Skyrocketing private health insurance costs are on track to consume ALL of our average household income by 2025. Even as premiums soar, insurance covers less of our health care costs every year. This is an industry on a death march.

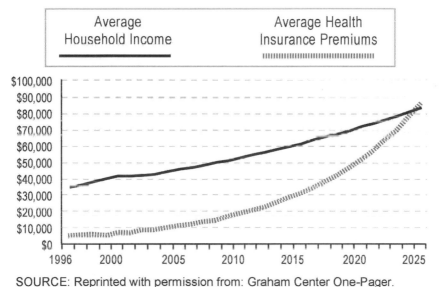

SOURCE: Reprinted with permission from: Graham Center One-Pager. Who will have health insurance in 2025? *Am Fam Physician* 72(10):2005,

What the Dying Insurance Industry Means For Most Americans

- Continued escalation of uncontrolled costs of health care
- Continued decline of employer-sponsored insurance
- Less insurance coverage for higher costs
- More insecurity over access to health care
- More corporate lobbying and disinformation as the industry fights a last-ditch battle for survival

"Geyman brings important news that everyone should recognize now, and will surely see in the coming years: that the private health insurance industry is obsolete, producing plans that are unaffordable when their coverage is good, and unusable when ordinary Americans can afford them. He shows how, in their death throes, they are becoming increasingly destructive. But unlike many other volumes, he shows that there is a way out, through a national single payer, non-profit fund that would cover all of us. Read it, and join the movement for universal care."

—Leonard Rodberg, PhD Professor of Urban Studies
Queens College, City University of New York

"There are two ways to heal the healthcare crisis in the United States. The first one doesn't work:

1. Pay more and more money to insurance companies to entice them to cover the uninsured and firmly regulate them so they stop denying healthcare to those who are already covered as well as the uninsured. Also stop their incursion into government-funded programs such as Medicaid, Medicare, SCHIP, and Vetcran's Healthcare.

2. A national single payer healthcare system that covers everyone, costs less money (because it cuts the insurance companies out of the control of our system) and provides more healthcare for every single person in the country.

John Geyman's book explains it all."

—Marilyn Clement,
National Coordinator Healthcare-NOW

"Congratulations on this very timely and helpful book. Keep up the great work!"

—David Satcher, M.D., PhD
16th Surgeon General of the United States
Director, National Center for Primary Care,
Morehouse School of Medicine

DO NOT RESUSCITATE

WHY THE HEALTH INSURANCE INDUSTRY IS DYING, AND HOW WE MUST REPLACE IT

John Geyman, M.D.

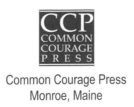

Common Courage Press
Monroe, Maine

ISBN 13 paperback: 978-1-56751-396-7
ISBN 13 hardback: 978-1-56751-397-4

Library of Congress Cataloging-in-Publication Data is available from publisher on request.

Common Courage Press
P.O. Box 702
121 Red Barn Road
Monroe, ME 04951
207-525-0900
fax: 207-525-3068

www.commoncouragepress.com
info@commoncouragepress.com

Second printing
Printed in Canada

Dedication

For the rapidly growing ranks of uninsured and underinsured
Americans without access to necessary health care.

May the day dawn when all Americans, as their birthright,
gain access to the health care that they need and deserve.

Contents

Tables and Figures

Acknowledgments

The support and encouragement of many colleagues have made this book possible. I am indebted to these colleagues for their constructive comments and suggestions through their peer review of selected chapters:

- Richard Deyo, MD, MPH, Kaiser Permanente Professor of Evidence-Based Family Medicine, Department of Family Medicine, Oregon Health and Science University

- David Gimlett, MD, long-time family physician and former Medical Director, Inter Island Medical Center, Friday Harbor, WA

- Larry Green, MD, Professor of Family Medicine and Director, Prescription for Health, University of Colorado Health Sciences Center

- Don McCanne, MD, past President of Physicians for a National Health Program and PNHP Senior Health Policy Fellow

- Charles North, MD, Clinical Director, Albuquerque Service Unit, Indian Health Service

- Roger Rosenblatt, MD, MPH, Professor of Family Medicine, University of Washington, Seattle

- John Saultz, MD, Professor and Chairman, Department of Family Medicine, Oregon Health Sciences University

- Joseph Scherger, MD, MPH, Professor of Family and Preventive Medicine, University of California, San Diego

Many sources of reference materials were especially helpful as this project progressed, especially reports from the Kaiser Family Foundation, the Commonwealth Fund, Public Citizen, the Center for Studying Health System Change, the Pew Research Center for the People and the Press, the Center for Responsive Politics, the National Academy of Social Insurance, the Medicare Rights Center, the

Medicare Payment Advisory Commission (MEDPAC), the Centers for Medicare-Medicaid Services (CMS), the Congressional Budget Office, and the General Accounting Office (GAO). Thanks are also due to the publishers and journals which granted permission to reprint or adapt materials as cited throughout the book.

As with my previous books, Virginia Gessner, my administrative assistant for over 30 years, meticulously converted handwritten manuscript through many drafts to final copy. Bruce Conway of Illumina Publishing, Friday Harbor, Washington brought his many skills to book design, cover and interior layout, preparation of all graphics and typesetting. And many thanks to Carolyn Acheson of Edmonds, Washington, for her very professional reader-helpful indexing of the book.

Finally, I am grateful to Greg Bates, Publisher at Common Courage Press for his discerning editorial expertise. His insightful suggestions have made this a better book. And as always, I thank Gene, my lovely wife and soul mate of 52 years, for her ongoing support, without which this work would never have seen the light of day.

Preface

Got Insurance?
Maybe, but How Much and for How Long?

The raging debate over how to pay for health insurance has missed a profoundly important fact: As big as it is, as tight of a grip as it has on American life, the health insurance industry is dying. Even industry insiders are worried about whether private insurance is sustainable. As far back as 1994, Bernard Tresnowski, as President of Blue Cross Blue Shield, issued the warning:[1]

> *"The good old days, when nobody really paid a lot of attention are gone. We're now front and center in the public policy sphere... What our future holds depends in many ways on our ability to continue to control the rate of increase of health care costs... It will be a real test over the next five to eight years as to whether the private sector indeed can produce the kind of results that would make health care more affordable."*

To understand how private health insurance could possibly be on the brink of extinction, we need to see our position today as a point on a trend line. Tracing the growth and evolution of the industry in this country makes clear not only where we are, but provides disturbing insights about where we are headed. As this book makes clear, the private health insurance industry is not sustainable, and has failed the public interest. Despite its claims, it does not provide more efficiency, value, and reliability than publicly-financed programs such as Medicare.

There is by now widespread consensus that the nation's health care system is broken and in urgent need of reform. There is also growing awareness among many health policy experts that incremental "reforms" will not resolve the inequities, access, cost, and quality problems of our unaccountable market-based system. The blame game is in full swing, with a circular firing squad targeting corporate stakeholders, employers, providers, or even patients themselves for their wasteful overuse of health care services. So far the private health insurance industry itself has not been called to account for its role in perpetuating our health care problems.

The U.S. is the only industrialized country around the world to base the financing of its health care system on a private insurance industry. Other nations have found one or another kind of social insurance necessary to provide universal coverage for their populations. Although our private health insurance was started and conducted in its early years on a not-for-profit basis, the industry has become largely for-profit and investor-owned over the last 40 years.

Though imposing by its size and $300 billion a year budget, the industry today profits by avoiding coverage of sick people, leaving them uninsured or underinsured while passing along coverage of the sick to increasingly beleaguered public safety net programs. Fragmentation of risk pools among more than 1,300 private insurers defeats the goal of insurance to provide coverage by sharing risk across a broad population. As the costs of health care continue to climb at rates two or three times faster than household incomes and costs of living, at least one-half of our population is having difficulty affording necessary health care. With 47 million Americans uninsured, the number of underinsured is soaring, and cost containment is still nowhere on the horizon.

The lessons we can glean from the track record of private health insurance in this country makes it easier to assess the confusing morass of incremental efforts to reform the industry and the system. If we are going to get to real solutions, we must grasp the ways by which the industry stands in the way of system reform. It will then be easier to create a road map to lasting health care reform. And it will also show why it has to be through a partnership between publicly-financed health insurance and a private delivery system.

This is a logical sequel to my five previous books on the health care system. The first dealt with the overall system,[2] followed by books on the corporate transformation of health care,[3] the uninsured and safety net,[4] privatization of Medicare,[5] and the corrosion of medicine.[6] All of the books focus on the commercial transformation of our health care system by corporate interests. *Do Not Resuscitate* carries that focus to the most fundamental aspect of our health care system—how we finance it—and maps out a vision and strategy for lasting reform.

I write this book for all the people who have no insurance, people who have insurance but are worried about what it covers or how to pay for it, people who are struggling with medical bills (insured or not), and people who have government insurance like Medicare or from the VA, but who worry about it being gnawed at by private interests. I write for business owners who can't afford to insure those they work with, or who are worried about competing against foreign businesses that don't have to shoulder that cost. I write for frustrated health professionals, frustrated patients, frustrated care givers and relatives of the ill. I write for those who have been sick and those who will be sick. And, of course, I write for the 535 members of Congress, in the hope that they will feel the growing pain of ordinary Americans over health care and will respond with real reform that most of the public has long supported. We are all in this together.

John P. Geyman, MD
May, 2008

References

1. Tresnowski B. President's Letter to BCBSA Plan CEOs. June 30, 1994, as cited in: Cunningham R., III, & Cunningham R. J., Jr. *The Blues: A History of the Blue Cross and Blue Shield System*, DeKalb, IL: Northern Illinois University Press, 1997, pp 250-1.
2. *Health Care in America: Can Our Ailing System Be Healed?* Woburn, Mass: Butterworth-Heinemann, 2002.
3. *The Corporate Transformation of Health Care: Can the Public Interest Still Be Served?* New York: Springer Publishing Company, 2004.
4. *Falling Through the Safety Net: Americans Confront the Perils of Health Insurance.* Monroe, ME: Common Courage Press, 2005.
5. *Shredding the Social Contract: The Privatization of Medicare.* Monroe, ME: Common Courage Press, 2006.
6. *The Corrosion of Medicine: Can the Profession Reclaim Its Moral Legacy?* Monroe, ME: Common Courage Press, 2007.

CHAPTER 1

In Sickness and in Wealth:
The Growth of a Monolithic Industry

"The high cost of health care has created a real burden
for the great financial middle class, composed of self-respecting
people who are too proud to accept free service and too poor to
be able to afford the costly private rooms, highly paid surgeons
and the expensive laboratory studies that have done so much to
take guesswork out of modern medicine and surgery."[1]

The above statement could well have been written today. Instead, it appeared in an editorial of the The *Saturday Evening Post* in 1926. The problems of limited access to health care and its increasing costs had led Theodore Roosevelt and the Progressive Party to make national health insurance (NHI) a platform plank in the presidential campaign of 1912, an effort finally defeated in 1917 by an alliance between employers and organized medicine.[2]

For almost 100 years in the United States, the subject of health insurance has been the target of intense debate and controversy and is still unresolved. Although the health care industry is now poised to surpass manufacturing as the leading industry in the U.S., with an enormous private health insurance industry playing a large part, the battle rages on over such basic issues as whether health insurance should be voluntary or compulsory, the roles of employers and the government, and whether health care is a basic human right or just another commodity to be bought and sold on the open market.

The problems of health care are complex. Soaring costs for new technology, increasing specialization, ever more complex and costly drugs, controversial interventions, new methods for early diagnosis, apportioning scarce resources from new machines to transplant organs, and the role of personal responsibility all compete as factors in our predicament. With all these factors in play, why is health insurance the core issue? As this book makes clear, how we insure against illness affects every aspect of the problem, from access to price, from efficient use of resources to the all-important sanctity of the doctor-patient relationship. No other issue in health care is as large a determinant of our collective well-being.

Because of its increasing unaffordability and decreasing coverage, health insurance has reached a crisis point. Concern has long been focused on the uninsured, yet they face new challenges. Where once the uninsured faced medical debt that was often free of interest, now, many debts are being managed by companies charging interest north of 14 percent, shooting monthly payments up fourfold or more. Even the insured face problems that emblazon the headlines. Bankruptcy due to medical bills has become a common problem, even when people have been employed and insured before they fell ill.

Understanding the evolution of our private financing system and its powerful interests is key to creating positive forces for change. It also reveals fascinating insights into what are now widely touted mantras of business: when there is competition, the customer always wins, and private enterprise is more efficient than government and non-profit sectors. The actual history of these ideas as played out in the insurance market is striking. In the early years, health insurance was made available on a not-for-profit basis through a quasi-public private partnership. In a second phase, trends transformed the mission and practices of the industry. Today's phase is marked by a growing disconnect of private health insurance from the needs of our population for adequate health coverage. Each phase contains important insights to better understand and respond to our current predicament.

The Early Years: A Quasi Public- Private Partnership of Socially-Oriented Insurance

Under different circumstances, the U.S. might well have adopted a national system of compulsory health insurance early in the 20th Century. Ten European countries, with Germany first, had adopted one or another form of compulsory health insurance between 1883 and 1913.[3] After England established a limited system in 1911, many American physicians believed that such a system was close to being enacted in this country.[4] Compulsory health insurance bills were introduced in 15 state legislatures between 1916 and 1920.[5] Congress held hearings in 1916 on a federal plan providing disability and sickness benefits.[6]

The social insurance committee of the American Medical Association (AMA) even passed this resolution in 1917.[7]

"the time is present when the profession should study earnestly to solve the questions of medical care that will arise under various forms of social insurance. Blind opposition, indignant repudiation, bitter denunciation of these laws is worse than useless: it leads nowhere and it leaves the profession in a position of helplessness as the rising tide of social development sweeps over it."

This resolution, however, encountered stiff opposition during further debate at the state level. The AMA soon reversed itself, digging in its heels against any compulsory health insurance, its steadfast policy to this day. When the U.S. entered World War I in 1917, national priorities changed abruptly, and public opinion shifted toward viewing compulsory health insurance as a foreign idea, tainted as un-American by its early connections with Germany, and the idea would not resurface until the Depression years.[8]

Local Initiatives Toward Prepayment

Although the start of health insurance in this country is often attributed to the emergence of a Blue Cross program for school teachers in Dallas, Texas in 1929, many other experiments had been taking place in earlier years to address problems in access and costs of health care. Congress established a sick fund for seamen in 1798 financed by a monthly payroll tax of 15 cents. St. Mary's Hospital in Saginaw, Michigan, sold certificates for $5.00 in the 1890s entitling their holders to a full range of hospital and physician services. Physicians in Grinnell, Iowa organized a hospital service plan in 1918. Local medical societies in King and Pierce Counties in Washington State established "industrial service bureaus," which could negotiate contracts between employers and employees on behalf of the physicians' organizations; by the end of 1917, four of five physicians in King County's Medical Society were involved in a plan covering 6,000 people. By 1919, 37 states had enacted workmen compensation programs. Prepaid group health care was available through company doctors in mine and mill towns in the Pacific Northwest and the Mesabi Range in Minnesota in the early years of the last century.[9]

As the country fell into the Depression at the close of the 1920s, the nation's hospitals were in dire economic straits, with more than one-third of all general hospital beds empty. Baylor's University Hospital in Dallas was one such hospital deeply in debt. Justin Ford Kimball, an attorney, university professor, and former school superintendent, was hired in 1929 to resuscitate the hospital's finances. He proceeded to design and implement a prepaid group hospital plan for over 1,300 Dallas teachers.

The Baylor Plan was the prototype upon which later Blue Cross plans were based. It provided free hospitalization for up to 21 days a year as well as coverage for operating room, laboratory and anesthesia services. Maternity benefits were limited to 50 percent of their costs and exclusions included pulmonary tuberculosis, smallpox, and chronic mental and nervous disorders. There was no third party; the hospital collected prepayments directly and assumed financial risk for the hospital care of the teachers' group.[10,11]

As the Great Depression deepened, many other new prepaid group programs sprouted up around the country for both hospital and medical care. Two hospitals in Sacramento, California, formed the first joint hospital prepayment plan in 1932; by 1935 the association included seven hospitals and almost 6,000 members.[12] Major multihospital Blue Cross plans were in operation in Durham, North Carolina, Washington, D.C. and Cleveland, Ohio by 1935; the Durham Plan was the first to include complete dependent coverage.[13] Drs. Donald Ross and Clifford Loos, after starting a prepaid contract practice in 1929 with employees of the Los Angeles Department of Water and Power, had enrolled 12,000 workers and 25,000 dependents in their plan by 1935, much to the alarm of the local medical society.[14]

Much of this activity was strongly opposed by organized medicine as a relentless march toward socialism. After six years of work, a major report was released in 1932 by the Committee on the Costs of Medical Care (CCMC). The group of 50 economists, physicians, public health professionals, administrators and scholars called for promotion of group practice and *voluntary* prepayment plans.[15] Dr. Morris Fishbein, then editor of The *Journal of the American Medical Association* (JAMA) wrote a scathing editorial in response to the CCMC's report, calling it "socialism and communism- inciting to revolution."[16] As President Franklin D. Roosevelt and Congress wrestled with how to cope with the country's economic woes, a compulsory system of national health insurance was dropped from New Deal programs of the mid-1930s, largely due to the strong opposition of organized medicine.[17]

The failure to include compulsory national health insurance during the New Deal years left a policy vacuum which Blue Cross plans, spurred on by the American Hospital Association (AHA), filled for a number of years on a not-for-profit socially-oriented basis. Leaders of newly emerged Blue Cross plans were successfully promoting themselves as alternatives to government-financed coverage of hospital care by arguing that its coverage would:

> ... "eliminate the demand for compulsory health insurance and stop the reintroduction of vicious sociological bills into the state legislature year after year—Blue Cross plans are a distinctly American institution, a unique combination of individual initiative and social responsibility. They perform a public service without public compulsion."[18]

They further marketed their plans in a 1939 press release as "a form of social insurance under non-governmental auspices, not merely a form of private insurance under non-profit auspices."[19]

At a 1937 meeting of the AHA, standards were adopted that would qualify as approved plans to carry the symbol of affiliation—a blue-colored cross with the AHA seal in the center. These standards provide a window on a different time, a day when concerns of investors were far distant, eclipsed by the needs of patients, hospitals and doctors. Historical documents can read as dusty reflections on less advanced times, but these nine standards provide a refreshing clarity on the timeless issues we struggle with today.[20]

- The corporate body should include representation of hospitals, the medical profession, and the general public.

- No private investors should provide money as stockholders or owners.

- Opportunities should be given for all hospitals in the community to participate in the hospitalization Plan, and subscribers should have free choice of hospital at times of illness.

- Benefits to subscribers should be guaranteed through service contracts with member hospitals, as opposed to cash indemnification contracts for hospital expenses.

- Annual subscription rates should be sufficient to remunerate hospitals properly for services rendered to subscribers.

- Uniform rates should be paid to participating hospitals for nominally similar services. Payments to hospitals should be based on the costs of services provided to subscribers in hospitals of the community, district, or region. This does not preclude... agreement by member hospitals to provide service at rates less than full operating costs.

- Employees of a nonprofit hospitalization Plan should be reimbursed by a salary as opposed to a commission basis. A private sales organization should not be given responsibility for promotion or administration on a percentage basis. Promotion and administration policies should be dignified in nature and consistent with the professional standards of the hospitals involved.

- Hospital services provided through hospitalization Plans should be determined by the practices of the hospitals and the wishes of the attending medical staffs in their communities.

- Hospitalization Plans should not interfere with existing relationships between physicians and hospitals, among physicians, or between physicians and patients.

The intent was to share risk across a broad risk pool in order to cover the sick and still keep premiums affordable. Emphasis was placed on service benefits of coverage instead of pre-determined fixed indemnity payments toward services received, as later offered by commercial carriers. By 1940 there were 39 state-based Blue Cross plans with an enrollment of more than 6 million people.[21]

Reaching back to those early days, it becomes clear that the history of American health insurance is the evolution from an effort to spread the risk, to today's focus on avoiding risk and maximizing profits. A look at the history between those times and today reveals how this tectonic shift occurred.

Rise of Employer-Sponsored Health Insurance

Although some companies were providing one or another kind of health care coverage in the 1930s, World War II was the main impetus for the rapid development of employer-sponsored insurance (ESI). A wartime economy brought the country out of the Depression and into a severe labor shortage. Unemployment rates dropped to little more than 1 percent. Federal wage and price controls made it difficult for employers to compete for workers by offering higher pay. Instead, the better capitalized employers turned to offering fringe benefits. IRS rulings allowed employers tax exemptions for the costs of health insurance, and these benefits were not taxable for employees.[22]

By the end of the war in 1945, about one-fourth of the population had some kind of health insurance, mostly for hospitalization.[23] In just one decade beginning in 1940, enrollment in private health insurance surged more than six-fold, from 12 million to more than 76 million. By 1950 a milestone had been reached: more than half of Americans were covered for the first time.[24]

Most of these new plans were Blue Cross plans, joined also by Blue Shield plans for coverage of physician services. Throughout the Great Depression, patients were having difficulty paying physicians out of pocket. The prototype Blue Shield plan was formed in 1939 as California Physicians' Service (CPS), later operating as Blue Shield of California, the country's first prepayment plan for medical services. The relationships between Blue Cross and Blue Shield plans varied widely from one part of the country to another, and were often contentious. Some Blue Shield plans were entirely independent of Blue Cross, while others cooperated on enrollment and some record-keeping but maintained separate Boards and staffs. James Stuart, who authored *The Blue Cross Story*, noted that "The history of Blue Cross and Blue Shield (Plans) has been one of undercover conflict."[25]

Despite the rapid growth of private ESI in the 1940s, battles were being waged, not just between many Blue Cross and Blue Shield plans, but also with new commercial insurers entering the market. As a loose confederation of diverse plans, Blue Cross Blue Shield (BCBS) found it a difficult challenge to compete against the for-profit commercial insurers, which brought an actuarial approach in bidding for contracts to provide indemnity coverage to large companies with plants and offices in several locations or whose businesses operated nationwide. Commercial insurers could relieve employers and unions of the burden of sorting through the maze of different rates and benefits offered by BCBS plans. Between 1940 and 1946, the number of group and individual policies held by commercial carriers nearly quadrupled to more than 14 million enrollees.[26]

Another part of an increasingly competitive marketplace was the emergence of new arrangements for health coverage by staff-model health maintenance organizations (HMOs) (See Glossary). Henry J. Kaiser established an early HMO in the shipyard industry in the 1940s, first as the Kaiser Foundation Health Plan and later as the Kaiser Permanente Health Plan. The Group Health Cooperative of Puget Sound was a similar not-for-profit staff model HMO started in the late 1940s.

Much of organized medicine continued to oppose these developments as beyond its direct control, even to the point of viewing their colleagues joining staff-model HMOs as socialists or communist sympathizers. But despite the turbulence of the health insurance marketplace at the close of the 1940s, one thing was clear. Voluntary pre-paid private health insurance was firmly entrenched across the country, and the threat of government-financed health care was put off for years to come. As Lawrence Brown, professor of health policy and management at Columbia University, recently observed: "The cultural die was cast: government's role in health coverage was officially confined to filling in the gaps of an otherwise robust private system."[27]

For a time at least, a quasi private-public system of socially-oriented health insurance was meeting the interests of employers, labor, and government for economic security concerning health care. That consensus was to change in years to follow.

Transformational Trends
After World War II

In the 60-plus years since the end of World War II, the private health insurance industry in the United States has been transformed from the quasi private-public partnership in its pioneering years to an enormous industry on a corporate mission of profit over service. The costs of health care and insurance premiums are soaring well above cost-of-living and family income levels, cost containment is nowhere on the horizon, and a majority of Americans are alarmed by a growing sense of insecurity about access and costs to necessary health care. A sea change has taken place in this country: Once, private health insurance had a mission to serve the public interest. Today, as will become clear later, the industry places its own self-interest above the public interest.

The Growth of Commercial Insurers

Recognizing the vast potential of the U.S. health insurance market, large numbers of for-profit commercial insurers entered the marketplace after World War II. Moving into the workplace market, they attracted many enrollees from not-for-profit Blues by offering lower-risk groups reduced premiums. Motivated largely by profits, commercial insurers worked aggressively to separate healthier enrollees from those expected to have higher health care costs, leaving the not-for-profit Blues with the challenge of dealing with adverse selection and competing for market share while covering sicker enrollees. Intense Darwinian competition soon developed in the health insurance market, fragmenting the risk pool into smaller and smaller parts.

Blue Cross plans were at a further disadvantage by providing full payments for standard benefits, such as the costs of hospitalization and ancillary services. By offering only limited indemnity coverage, commercial insurers could insulate themselves from rising costs of hospital care and undercut Blues' premiums.[28] Commercial carriers also gained market share by offering "major medical", catastrophic coverage especially attractive to higher-income enrollees which typically provided coverage up to $10,000 for such expenses as outpatient care, diagnostic and laboratory tests, drugs, and convalescent care. By 1959, 22 million Americans had some form of major medical coverage.[29] Between 1950 and 1960, the number of Americans with health insurance grew from 77 to 132 million, with the commercial insurers gaining the largest share of this growth. By 1961, there were 800 commercial carriers with 40 million individual enrollees.[30]

The Shift from Spreading Risk to Avoiding It: Underwriting and Experience Rating

Winning over this large number of new enrollees to the commercial insurers altered the competitive landscape and heightened the focus on profit. In response to fierce competition in the health insurance market in the 1950s, the Blues were under pressure to compromise their traditional service mission and experiment with experience rating and indemnity coverage, especially in the individual non-group market.

In the early years of the private health insurance in this country as pioneered by Blue Cross plans, community rating was the norm, whereby risk was shared across all enrollees in the covered population at the same premium. Coverage was typically offered to all comers (guaranteed issue). Medical underwriting, by which insurers charge higher premiums for enrollees considered to be at higher risk for illness, was considered unethical.

All of this changed after World War II. Experience rating, by which insurers increase premiums based upon the claims made by enrollees and avoid high-risk individuals and groups, has been the industry norm for many years.

From the 1950s on, commercial insurers often required physical examinations before providing coverage, one commercial plan set an enrollment age limit at age 50, and most limited conversion from group to individual coverages. By 1959, more than two-thirds of Blue Cross plans practiced experience rating by such requirements as age limits, requiring applicants to be employed, or not covering maternity care for the first ten months after enrollment.[31] A 2004 report of an historical data set from 1957 concluded that:

> *"Based on the evidence presented here showing that the Blues did suffer from adverse selection in the individual market, and based on later claims that the Blues were unable to compete with experience rated plans, it seems likely that Blue*

Cross and Blue Shield may have ultimately faced three choices: succumb to the adverse selection death spiral, experience rate their policies to more effectively compete with commercial firms, or ask for help from state insurance regulators. "[32]

Fast forward to 1982: After many years of strained relations between them, Blue Cross and Blue Shield agreed to merge. They did this partly to protect their market share and to gain political strength to represent their views and head off government intervention. [33]

By the 1990s, most of the health insurance industry had converted to experience rating, with the Blues mostly forced to abandon community rating and mimic the practices of their commercial competition. The implications of these dynamics were not lost on Blue Cross Blue Shield. As Thomas Kinser, chief operating officer of the Blue Cross Blue Shield Association (BCBSA) lamented in 1992:

> *"With modern electronic data processing technology and new rating methods, these cherry-picking companies can   under the current rules [and] with full blessing of insurance commissions—find good risks, raise rates enormously if they get claims at the end of the first year, and have a pool of business that they [profit from]... But they are not looking for stability of relationships with customers, predictable financing, and good community health systems.* "[34]

While some higher-risk people were insured at high premium rates, they were the lucky ones. Many others were denied coverage altogether. Risks used by commercial insurers to deny coverage in the early 1990s included.[35]

- Acquired immunodeficiency syndrome (AIDS)
- Ulcerative colitis
- Cirrhosis of liver
- Diabetes mellitus
- Leukemia
- Schizophrenia
- Hypertension (uncontrolled)

- Emphysema
- Stroke
- Obesity (severe)
- Angina (severe)
- Coronary artery disease
- Epilepsy
- Lupus
- Alcoholism/drug abuse

Table 1.1 compares denial rates for individual applicants in 2001.[36]

Table 1.1

Denial Rates for Individual Health Insurance Applicants with Specified Health Conditions/Histories, 2001

Condition/ history	Denial rate % (60 applications)	Number affected by health condition
Seasonal allergies (hay fever)	8%	36 million
History of knee injury	12%	5 million
Asthma	15%	17 million
Breast cancer survivor	43%	8.4 million*
Depression	23%	19 million
Hypertension,overweight, smoker	55%	64 million (hypertension) 69 million (obesity) 47 million (smokers)
HIV/AIDS	100%	800,000-900,000

Source: Pollitz K., et al. How accessible is individual health insurance for consumers in less-than-perfect health? Menlo Park, CA: Henry J. Kaiser Family Foundation, Reprinted with permission. * Survivors of cancer of all types.

Managed Care

As a new effort to contain health care costs, the rapid growth of managed care in the 1980s and 1990s added further complexity and turmoil to the health care marketplace while disrupting many relationships between patients, providers (the new-jargon for physicians and other health professionals), and insurers. Managed care altered methods of payment for health care services from fee-for-service (FFS) to prospective payment based on capitation, or reimbursement to providers based on the number of individuals enrolled in a health plan (See also Glossary). It also brought increasing fragmentation and bureaucracy, less choice of provider and hospital, and more frequent denial of services for physicians and their patients. Figure 1.1 shows a wide spectrum among health plans in terms of choice and cost control.

The Blues were slower to join the managed care movement than commercial carriers, but by the early 1990s had actively diversified their products. By 1995, Blue Plans had enrolled 8 million people in HMO programs, passed Kaiser Permanente as the industry's largest

Figure 1.1

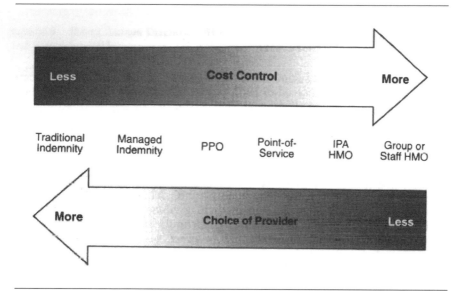

Source: Reprinted with permission from Dowling WL. The future of managed care. Presented at 28th Annual Advances in Family Practice and Primary Care course. Seattle, WA; University of Washington, September 14, 2000.)

HMO purveyor, and claimed 22 million enrollees in their preferred provider organizations (PPOs) and point-of-service (POS) plans (defined in the Glossary).[37]

Toward For-Profit and Investor Ownership: Whose Health Insurance Is It Now?

As the traditionally not-for-profit Blues lost more enrollees to commercial carriers, they were left with higher-risk enrollees requiring increasing premiums to stay afloat, in turn further threatening their market share. A death march was in progress, and the Blues found themselves under growing public scrutiny. A three-year investigation of Blue Cross Plans led to a book published by Yale University Press in 1976 *Blue Cross: What Went Wrong?*, which concluded that "examination of Blue Cross reveals not so much a system out of control as a system that is quite effectively designed to meet needs and interests that are not the needs and interest of those who use and pay for health services."[38]

Ten years later, the transition from a public service mission to a business focused on serving the interests of investors was so far along that two branches of the U.S. government took notice. The U.S. General Accounting Office (GAO) found "more similarities than differences between the Blues and commercial carriers" concerning their approach to high-risk individuals, and the IRS noted that "the significant differences between non-profit and for-profit insurers that may have justified the initial tax exemptions have been eroded by competitive developments."[39] Soon afterward, Congress passed the Tax Reform Act of 1986 which taxed Blues' net income at 20 percent (lower than the 34 percent commercial rate, but subject to some restrictions).[40]

Under these mounting pressures, the unity of BCBS plans was being seriously challenged. Three of four BCBS plans believed in 1993 that the non-profit license standard should be dropped, and new licensing standards were adopted in 1994 without that requirement. [41] In subsequent years, an increasing number of Blues Plans became publicly traded investor-owned corporations. By 2005, one-half of the nation's Blue Cross plans had been consolidated and converted into for-profit companies.[42]

Limited Regulatory Oversight

Most regulation of the insurance industry was ceded to the states when Congress passed the McCarren-Ferguson Act in 1945. Since then, we have seen a maze of limited industry-friendly regulations varying widely from one state to another. The insurance industry maintains the largest lobbying presence in state capitols across the country, with frequent revolving door relationships and conflicts of interest with state legislatures. In Virginia, for example, 26 legislators had ties to the insurance industry during the November 2000 election campaign, when HMOs successfully fought off, by a narrow margin, patients' rights legislation that would have permitted patients to sue their HMOs.[43]

In an average state, about one-third of the insured population has insurance that is subject to state regulatory agencies. All federal programs, including Medicare, Medicaid, the Veterans Administration, and other plans are exempt from state regulations. The Employee Retirement Income and Security Act of 1974 (ERISA) also exempted all self-funded employee benefit programs. By 1990, more than two-thirds of American companies, including virtually all of the largest, had gained this exemption by self-insuring.[44, 45] Even where state regulations do apply to health insurance, these regulations are often permissive to industry. A national survey in 2000, for example, found that 39 states do not require private health insurers to offer prescription drug coverage and that lifetime dollar limits are allowed in most states.[46] In addition, many insurers game the system by establishing administrative bases in states with lax regulations while conducting business through out-of-state groups.[47]

Consolidation and the Growing Power of Insurers

Another major transformational change affecting the health insurance industry is the growing pace of consolidation in recent years. As the largest of all private health insurers, Wellpoint was formed in 2004 through the merger of Anthem and Wellpoint Health Networks. Between 1995 and 2005, more than 400 mergers took place involving insurers and managed care organizations. As a result of these mergers and consolidation, the industry gains new leverage and negotiating power with providers and patients. A recent example was the all-cash purchase of Sierra Health Services by Minnesota-based United Health Group.

This merger sent off alarm bells and opposition by the AMA, which estimates that United Health will now control 78 percent of the HMO market in Nevada and 95 percent of the HMO market in the Las Vegas-Paradise area.[48] The GAO has found a steady increase in market share among private insurers in the small group market, primarily served by BCBS plans. The combined median market share of the largest small group carrier increased from 33 percent to 43 percent from 2002 to 2004.[49]

Decline of Employer-Sponsored Health Insurance (ESI)

There is growing recognition in recent years that ESI is an unsatisfactory and unsustainable way to finance the bulk of the nation's health care system.[50-52] After all, it was an accident of history organized rapidly in the wartime economy of World War II, hardly a well-planned financing system upon which to build a large part of the overall economy. By 2005, ESI covered only about 56 percent of employees working more than 20 hours a week, down from more than 70 percent in 1980. Those workers still with coverage find their benefits unraveling as employers shift from defined-benefits to a defined-contribution approach and require increased cost-sharing by employees.[53]

ESI arose in another age when American business was dominant, had few concerns about global competition, and when labor unions were strong. That time has long since passed. Many industries, as illustrated by the auto industry, are at a competitive disadvantage in the new global economy with countries which have publicly-financed health care. A growing number of U.S. employers are slashing coverage of their employees' health care costs. [54]

Shift to Consumer-Directed Health Care (CDHC)

Even as health care costs continue to surge well beyond cost-of-living and family income levels, recent years have seen the responsibility for cost control placed directly on patients themselves. Many employers and conservatives in government are joining what Jacob Hacker, Professor of Political Science at Yale University calls the Personal Responsibility Crusade in his recent book *The Great Risk Shift: The Assault on American Jobs, Families, Health Care, and Retirement and How You Can Fight Back.*[55]

The insurance industry has welcomed this new trend by rolling out a variety of stripped-down limited benefit plans.[56] Insurers are carving out profitable new niches in the market, targeted at healthier enrollees. Examples include high-deductible health insurance (HDHI) plans with deductibles up to $10,000,[57] and short-term policies which exclude any pre-existing condition and offer no continuing protection, and policies with capped benefits.[58]

These policies further fragment an already hypersegmented risk pool, defeating the basic principle of insurance to share risks broadly. By offering these kinds of incomplete policies at affordable premiums, insurers create the illusion of coverage to employers and enrollees alike. Instead, enrollees with any significant illness are likely to find the costs of necessary health care unaffordable and many who remain healthy are worried about being vulnerable to huge expenses if they get sick.

Privatization of Public Programs

Still another major trend, ironically enough, which has transformed the private health insurance industry in this country is the increasing privatization of public programs. Both Medicare and Medicaid have provided insurers with lucrative new markets. The Medicare Prescription Drug, Improvement, and Modernization Act of 2003 (MMA) opened up vast markets by requiring the new prescription drug benefit to be managed through the private sector. Traditional Medicare was not permitted to administer the new Part D drug benefit, and the government was prohibited from negotiating drug prices. Instead, the MMA required that private managed care organizations and pharmacy benefit managers administer the benefit, with generous subsidies from the government. Despite the failure of private Medicare + Choice plans to either contain costs or maintain reliable coverage during the 1990s, the MMA re-authorized private Medicare HMO-PPOs under the banner of Medicare Advantage, again with government overpayments much higher than the costs of traditional Medicare.[59]

Humana's experience shows just how profitable the drug benefit can be. After grabbing the largest market share of the Part D drug benefit by offering low initial premiums, premiums were later hiked in bait and switch fashion: In 2005, Humana's return to investors soared to 83 percent.[60, 61] In 2006, Humana's fourth-quarter net income more than doubled to $155 million, while its pretax profit from government business more than tripled.[62]

Meanwhile, many states have contracted out much of their Medicaid programs to private companies, again without a track record of greater efficiency or reliability and with little accountability. Two examples illustrate how far some private managed care companies are willing to go to cut costs of care and maximize their profits. In New Jersey, private Medicaid companies enrolled large numbers of low-income families and then rejected up to 30 percent of their claims for hospital care.[63] In Massachusetts, private Medicaid contractors have pocketed capitation income while holding "covered" children, after voluntary admissions, in locked wards of psychiatric hospitals without medical indications and with minimal treatment.[64] According to an investigative report by the *Boston Sunday Globe*, one staff member

admitted that these children
were placed in locked wards
"because the census was
down."[65]

Privatization of public
programs has clearly been a
financial bonanza for private
insurers. One example: a private equity fund cashed out
a $220 million investment in
WellCare purchased in 2002
for $870 million in 2006. An-
nual revenues of the four fastest growing Medicaid HMOs
quadrupled between 2001
and 2006, as shown in Figure
1.2.[66]

Figure 1.2

Taking Over the Market

Combined annual revenue of four of the fastest-growing Medicaid HMOs:

$12 Billion

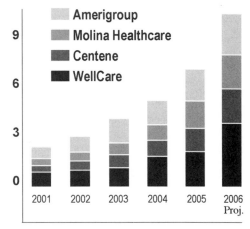

SOURCE: the companies; Goldman Sachs

The Industry Today:
A Growing Disconnect From Health Care Needs

The American health care system has two enormous costs that other countries with government financed health insurance don't have. The first is the profit that companies make for private investors, as discussed above. Table 1.2 shows the six leading U.S. health insurance and managed care companies by profits, medical-loss ratios, total return to investors, and size of workforce. Of particular interest are the striking increases in profits of some companies from 2004 to 2005, as well as the swelling ranks of their workforces.[67, 68]

Aside from lining the pockets of investors, the second enormous drag on our health care dollar is lower efficiency of private insurers compared to publicly-financed insurance. Countries with government-financed health insurance are much more efficient than private financing. Canada, for example, while spending little more than one-half the amount per capita on health care than the U.S., covers all Canadians with a comparatively small administrative workforce and overhead. In contrast, the U.S. has some 1,300 private companies in its national trade group, America's Health Insurance Plans (AHIP). With a workforce 10 to 25 times larger than Canada's single-payer system, [69] the industry consumes more than $300 billion in spending each year[70] and still leaves 47 million Americans uninsured and tens of million other citizens underinsured.

Despite the claims of the industry that it is the backbone of financing for U.S. health care, the evidence points in the opposite direction. With their priorities on profits and return to their shareholders, private insurers cherry-pick low-risk enrollees from higher-risk groups and individuals to keep their "medical loss" ratios below 80 percent if possible (ie., keep at least 20 percent of premium dollar income). Insurers understand that 5 percent of people account for 50 percent of total annual health spending, 10 percent for 72 percent and 20 percent for 90 percent.[71] Most of these people can be readily excluded by sharp medical underwriting and experience rating. Much of the workforce effort and administrative overhead of private insurers is focused on three tasks designed to avoid paying for medical costs: trying to avoid covering people who are high risk (and would be costly), denying many claims of people who do get sick, and reunderwriting (usually once a

Table 1.2

LEADING HEALTH INSURANCE AND MANAGED CARE COMPANIES, 2006

Industry Rank	Company	Profits $Million	Rank	% Change from 2004	Medical-Loss Ratio	Total Return to Investors	Employees	% Change from 2004
1	United Health Group	3,300	1	28	78.6%	41%	55,000	38%
2	Wellpoint	2,464	2	157	80.6%	39%	42,000	11%
3	Aetna	1,635	3	(27)	76.9%	51%	28,200	6%
4	Cigna	1,625	4	13	82.3%	37%	28,000	(2%)
5	Humana	308	5	10	83.2%	83%	18,700	36%
6	Health Net	230	6	439	83.9%	79%	9,131	8%

Sources: Fortune 1,000. Ranked within industries. 28 HealthCare: Insurance and Managed Care. F-52. FORTUNE APRIL 17, 2006. Medical-loss ratios from Company 10-K, year-end filings with the Securities and Exchange Commission.

year) with premium hikes for sick enrollees with higher claims.

Growth in administrative overhead isn't driven by a need to cover more patients. Between 2000 and 2005, although the number of Americans with private insurance dropped by 1 percent, the private insurance workforce grew by one-third.[72] Over the last three decades, the ranks of administrative personnel have grown by 25 times the numbers

Figure 1.3

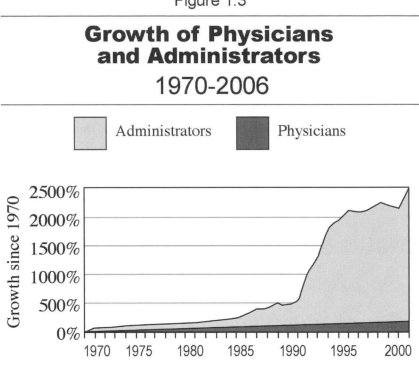

Growth of Physicians
and Administrators
1970-2006

SOURCE: Reprinted with permission from: Woolhandler S. & Himmelstein DU. The National Health Program Slide-show Guide, Center for National Health Program Studies, Cambridge, Mass, 2006.

of physicians, as shown in Figure 1.3.

Despite all its claimed importance as the main way in which U.S. health care is financed, the private health insurance industry plays a much smaller role than public financing. Actually, private health insurance through ESI now accounts for only 35 percent of total health care spending.[73] Public programs finance the majority of annual health care costs. Thomas Selden, economist at the federal Agency for Healthcare Research and Quality (AHRQ) estimates that the government finances

60 percent of the nation's annual health care bill, including direct pay-ments for services as well as subsidies for tax exemptions. Princeton's health economist Uwe Reinhardt factors in another 5 percent for the federal mandate that hospitals provide free care to the uninsured.[74]

Having reviewed the historic shift from mission-based nonprofit health insurance that spreads the risk across the healthy and the sick to a for-profit system that avoids risk, shuts out those who need insur-ance, and concentrates profit and power, the question arises: What can we expect next? Two trends are rolling forward that suggest that the days of industry profits from coverage of a declining population are numbered. Employer Sponsored Insurance, ESI, is on a steady decline. The bulk of the private health insurance business is still through ESI. Just 17 million Americans (6.7 percent of the population) get private insurance individually. But individual applicants for coverage face a rough time. Many applicants for individual coverage are either turned down at the outset or, if covered, soon find their premiums unafford-able.[75] A 2006 study by the Commonwealth Fund found that one-third of applicants could not find needed individual coverage, and that for 58 percent of adults shopping for coverage, it was unaffordable.[76] These twin dynamics, declining ESI and an individual market that can't take up the slack because it is becoming less affordable, are turning the U.S. private health insurance industry toward government programs for its future growth.[77]

Just how fast are these dynamics moving? The increasing unaf-fordability of private health insurance has become the Achilles heel of the entire industry, now broadly impacting middle America. The average family premium for employer-based coverage rose to $11,500 in 2006, an increase of 87 percent between 2000 and 2006.[78] By 2025, annual health insurance premiums are projected to consume the *entire* average family income, clearly a crisis well before then (Figure 1.4).[79] Already, household income has been relatively flat for the last two de-cades while the level of household debt is soaring (now over $100,000 compared to median family income of $41,000).[80] In 2003, one-third of Americans had medical expenses that were at least 20 percent of their family income, while more than 10 percent had expenses exceed-ing their entire income.[81]

What does this trend mean for the public? American frustration over health care has risen to such a fever pitch that, together with the

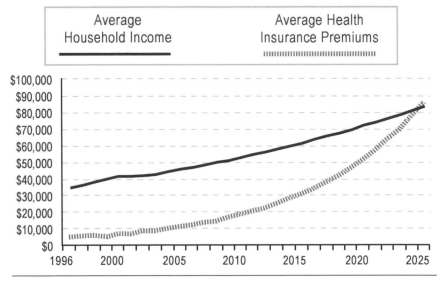

Figure 1.4

Annual Health Insurance Premiums and Household Income, 1996 to 2025

Source: Reprinted with permission from: Graham Center One-Pager.
Who will have health insurance in 2025? *Am Fam Physician* 72(10):2005.

economy, it has actually eclipsed the unpopular war in Iraq as a leading issue in the 2008 election. A new flurry of incremental "reform" proposals is being bandied about to assure universal access (to health insurance). That is not the biggest problem, though, because most of the effort to expand the number of uninsured ends up as underinsurance, providing little security against the costs of necessary health care. The rate of bankruptcies related to medical bills has risen to an all-time high. Of the 1 million Americans bankrupted each year as a result of medical bills, three of four are not only employed but also insured before becoming sick.[82]

A growing part of the population is losing access to basic health care as financial barriers continue to rise. According to a 2007 report, the percentage of primary care physicians not accepting new patients by expected payment source has grown to 45 percent for charity, 31 percent for capitated private insurance, 29 percent for Medicaid, and 20 percent for Medicare.[83] The Institute of Medicine has calculated that

8 million uninsured Americans with chronic disease have increased morbidity and worse outcomes, and that 18,000 people die premature and preventable deaths each year.[84]

Whither Private Health Insurance?

Given these marked transformational changes over the past six decades in the U.S., what can we anticipate for the future of the private health insurance industry? It is pricing itself beyond the reach of a declining private market, even as it seeks out a broader, subsidized role in public programs. All incremental approaches to prop up the industry in recent years have failed to resolve the country's increasing problems of access and cost of health care.

The much more important question, however, is what is to become of U.S. health care? Can the nation develop enough consensus and political will to confront its increasingly serious system problems? As various reform alternatives come under consideration, a central question arises: Has the private health insurance industry outlived its role as a financing mechanism for U.S. health care?

This book will consider these questions with a goal toward a better understanding of the options before us. There is widespread denial that the heath care system is as sick as it is, and market interests keep telling us that markets can resolve our problems. This "reassurance," however, has already been discredited, and the health care system is in a deepening hole. At this point, we need to recall the Old Farmer's Advice, "if you find yourself in a hole, the first thing to do is to stop diggin!"

As a start toward exploring the status of the private health insurance industry, we'll turn in the next chapter to a profile of the three largest insurers which dominate the industry.

References

1.   Editorial on health care costs in a 1926 issue of *Saturday Evening Post* as cited in: Proceedings of Spring Meeting of Society of Actuaries, Spring 2007, Seattle, Wash.

2.   Somers A.R. & Somers H.M. *Health and Health Care: Policies in Perspectives*. Germantown, MD: Aspen Systems Corporation, 1977, pp 179-

80.

3.   Starr P. *The Social Transformation of American Medicine*. New York: Basic
        Books, 1982, pp. 252-3.
4.   Numbers R. L. *Almost Persuaded: American Physicians and Compulsory
        Health Insurance*, 1912-1920. Baltimore: Johns Hopkins Press, 1978.
5.   Burrow J.G. *AMA: Voice of American Medicine*. Baltimore: Johns Hopkins
        Press, 1963, pp 144-5.
6.   Ibid #2.
7.   Ibid #5.
8.   Cunningham R.C.III & Cunningham R.M.,Jr. *The Blues: A History of the Blue
        Cross and Blue Shield System*. DeKalb, IL: The Northern Illinois University
        Press, 1997, pp 35-6.
9.   Ibid 8, p 8-9, 36.
10.   Stuart J.E. *The Blue Cross Story: An Informal Biography of the Voluntary
        Nonprofit Prepayment Plan for Hospital Care*. Chicago: BCBSA archives.
        Photocopied typescript, circa 1966, p 19.
11.   Blue Cross and Blue Shield of Texas. *Advance*, June 1989. Corporate
        periodical, p 6.
12.   Ibid #10, pp 24-5.
13.   Ibid #10, pp 29-30.
14.   MacColl W.A. Group Practice and Prepayment of Medical Care. Washington,
        D.C.: Public Affairs Press, 1966, p 12.
15.   Committee on the Costs of Medical Care (CCMC). Medical Care for the
        American People: The Final Report. Chicago: University of Chicago Press,
        1932, pp 7, 41.
16.   Campion F.D. *The AMA and U.S. Health Policy Since 1940*. Chicago: Chicago
        Review Press, 1984, p 117.
17.   Ibid #2, pp 266-70.
18.   Rothman D. J. The public perception of Blue Cross, 1935-1965. *J Health
        Polit, Policy Law* 16(4):671, 1991.
19.   Heidinger F.R. *The Social Role of Blue Cross as a Device for Financing the
        Costs of Hospital Care: An Evaluation*. Iowa City, Iowa: Graduate Program in
        Hospital and Health Administration, University of Iowa, 1966, 20-21.
20.   Ibid #8, pp 29-30.
21.   Somers H.M. & Somers A.R. *Doctors, Patients, and Health Insurance*.
        Washington, D.C.: The Brookings Institution, 1961, p 548.
22.   Ibid #2, pp 109-11.
23.   Labor Research Association. *Labor Fact Book 8*. New York: International
        Publishers, 1947.
24.   Hacker J.S. *The Great Risk Shift: The Assault on American Jobs, Families,
        Health Care, and Retirement* and *How You Can Fight Back*. New York:
        Oxford University Press, 2006, p 145.
25.   Ibid #10, p 128.
26.   Ibid #21,
27.   Brown L.D. The more things stay the same, the more they change. The odd

interplay between government and ideology in the recent political history of the U.S. health-care system. In: Stevens R.A., Rosenberg C.E. & Burns L.R. (eds). *History and Health Policy in the United States*: *Putting the Past Back In*. New Brunswick, NJ: Rutgers University Press, 2006, p 45.

28. Ibid #8, pp 92-3.
29. Ibid #26, pp 281-2.
30. Andrews C. *Profit Fever*: *The Drive to Corporatize Health Care and How to Stop It*. Monroe, ME: Common Courage Press, 1995, pp 3-8.
31. Thomasson M.A. Early evidence of an adverse selection dealth spiral? The case of Blue Cross and Blue Shield. *Explorations in Economic Society* 41:313-28, 2004.
32. Ibid #31, p 327.
33. Ibid #8, pp 194-5.
34. Ibid #8, p 216.
35. Light D.W. The practice and ethics of risk-rated health insurance. JAMA 267:2503, 1992.
36. Pollitz K., et al. How accessible is individual health insurance for consumers in less-than-perfect health? Menlo Park, CA: Henry J. Kaiser Family Foundation, 2002.
37. Ibid #8, p 251.
38. Law S., et al. *Blue Cross: What Went Wrong?* 2nd ed. New Haven: Yale University Press, 1976, p 160.
39. U.S. General Accounting Office, *Health Insurance: Comparing Blue Cross and Blue Shield Plans with Commercial Insurers*, 1986, esp. pp 2-3.
40. Ibid #8, p 215.
41. Ibid #8, p 247.
42. Schramm C. The diseconomies of Blue Cross conversion. Washington, D.C.: Alliance for Advancing Non-profit Healthcare, February 2005.
43. Renzulli D. & The Center for Public Integrity. *Capitol offenders: How private interests govern our states*. Washington, D.C.: Center for Public Integrity, pp 94-5, 2002.
44. Iglehart J.K. State regulation of managed care: Interview with NAIC President Joseph Musser. *Health Aff (Millwood)* 16:36, 1997.
45. Ibid #8, p 218.
46. Bolin J. N., Buchanan R. J. & Smith S. R. State regulation of private health insurance: prescription drug benefits, experimental treatments, and consumer protection. *Am J Manage Care* 8:977, 2002.
47. Terhune C. Insurers avoid state regulations by selling via groups elsewhere. *The Wall Street Journal*, April 9, 2002, p A20.
48. AMA. AMA asks Justice Department to block takeover of Sierra Health Services, March 19, 2007.
49. U.S. General Accounting Office (GAO). *Private Health Insurance: Number and market Share of Carriers in the Small Group Health Insurance Market in 2004*. Letter to the Committee on Small Business and Entrepreneurship, United States Senate, October 13, 2005.

50.   Taylor H. How and why the health insurance system will collapse. *Health Aff (Millwood)* 21, 195:2002.
51.   Kuttner R. The American health care system: Health insurance coverage. N *Engl J Med* 340:163, 1999.
52.   Fuchs V. What's ahead for health insurance in the United States? *N Engl J Med* 346:13, 2002.
53.   Mishel L., Bernstein J., & Allegretto S. *The State of Working America 2004/2005*. Ithaca: Cornell University Press, 2005, data available online at www,epinet.org/content.cfm/datazone_dznational.
54.   Nocera J. Resolving to re-imagine health costs. *New York Times*, November 18, 2006:B1.
55.   Ibid #24, p 149.
56.   Robinson J.C. The end of managed care. JAMA 285 (20):2622-8,2001
57.   Robinson J.C. consumer -directed health insurance: the next generation. An interview with John Rowe. *Health Affairs Web Exclusive*, December 13, 2005
58.   Chaker A. M. A pinch hit on health coverage. *The Wall Street Journal*, May 7, 2001, p D6.
59.   Bodenheimer T. The dismal failure of Medicare privatization. Senior Action Network, San Francisco, June, 2003, p 1.
60.   Krasner J. Insurer hits millions of seniors with drug cost hike. *Boston Globe*, December 31, 2006.
61.   Fortune 1,000 ranked by industries. Health care: Insurance and managed care. F-52. *Fortune* April 17, 2006.
62.   Zhang J., & Fuhrmans U. Government pays growing share of health costs. *New York Times*, February 21, 2007:A1.
63.   Freudenheim M. Some concerns thrive on Medicaid patients. The *New York Times*, February 19, 2003, p C1.
64.   Wolfe S. M. Unhealthy partnership: How Massachusetts and its managed care contractor shortchange troubled children. *Public Citizen Health Research Group Health Letter*, 17(2):1, 2001.
65.   Kong D. & O"Neill G. Locked wards open door to booming business. *Boston Sunday Globe*, May 11, 1997, A1.
66.   Martinez B. Healthy industry. In Medicaid, private HMOs take a big, and lucrative role. *Wall Street Journal*, November 15, 2006:A1.
67.   Ibid #61.
68.   Bethely J.G. Health plans make more, spend less in 2005. *American Medical News*, March 6, 2006
69.   Woolhandler S., Campbell T., & Himmelstein D. U. Costs of health care administration in the United States and Canada. *N Engl J Med* 349:768, 2003.
70.   Kleinke J. D. *Oxymorons: The Myths of the U.S. Health Care System*. San Francisco: Jossey-Bass, 2001, p 192.
71.   Stoll K. & Denker P. What's wrong with tax-free savings accounts for health care? Issue Brief. *Families USA*. Washington, D.C.: November 2003.
72.   Krugman P. The world of U.S. health care economics is downright scary.

Seattle Post Intelligencer September 26, 2006:B1.

73. Woolhandler S., & Himmelstein D. U. Paying for national health insurance—and not getting it. *Health Aff (Millwood)* 21(4):88-98, 2002.

74. Gross D. National health care? We're halfway there. *New York Times*, December 3, 2006.

75. Turnbull N.C., & Kane N. M. Insuring the healthy or insuring the sick? The dilemma of regulating the individual health insurance market. The Commonwealth Fund, New York: February 2005.

76. Collins S.R., Kriss J.L., Davis K., Doty M.M., et al. Squeezed: Why rising exposure to health care costs threatens the health and financial well-being of American families. The Commonwealth Fund. New York, September, 2006.

77. Ibid #62.

78. Barry P., & Basler B. Healing our system. *AARP Bulletin*, 48(3), March 2007, p 2.

79. Graham Center One-Pager. Who will have health insurance in 2025? *Am Fam Physician* 72(10):1989, 2005.

80. Henderson N. Greenspan's mixed legacy: America prospered during the Fed chiefs tenure, but built up massive debt. *Washington Post National Weekly Edition*. January 30— February 5, 2006.

81. Ibid #24, p 142.

82. Himmelstein D.U., Warren E., Thorne D. & Woolhandler S. Illness and injury as contributors to bankruptcy. *Health Affairs Web Exclusive* W5-63, 2005.

83. Communicable Disease Center(CDC). MMWR. QuickStats: Percentage of office-based primary care physicians who did not accept new patients, by expected payment source. National Ambulatory Medical Care Survey, United States, 2003-2004, March 16, 2007.

84. Committee on the Consequences of Uninsurance: *Hidden costs, value lost: Uninsurance in America.* Institute of Medicine. Washington, D.C.: National Academy Press, 2003.

CHAPTER 2

The Big Three and the Three M's: Mergers, Market Share, and Medical-Loss Ratios

Three giant private health insurers have come to dominate the industry in this country, collectively covering about 75 million Americans. A brief profile of each of these companies provides a thumbnail sketch of a turbulent market in which mergers, market share, and medical-loss ratios are the coin of the realm. The private insurance industry sees whatever premium revenue that is actually spent on care of patients as a loss, hence the term "medical loss ratio" (MLR) (formerly called "medical cost ratio") or that portion of the premium dollar spent on direct medical care. As we will soon find, reviewing the operations of the industry from the standpoints of mergers, market share, and MLRs shows to what extent the industry is now driven to corporate profits rather than serving its enrollees.

Wellpoint Inc.

As the nation's largest private health insurer, Indianapolis-based Wellpoint covers about 34 million people in 14 states. It was formed in 2004 when Anthem Inc. bought Thousand Oaks, California-based Wellpoint Health Networks, Inc. Most of its subsidiaries are BCBS companies, including Blue Cross of California, Blue Cross Blue Shield of Georgia, Blue Cross Blue Shield of Missouri, and Wellchoice, parent of the largest insurer in New York State, for-profit Empire Blue Cross-Blue Shield. According to a 2007 Hoover's Inc. report of key financials, Wellpoint, Inc. gained a one-year growth in net income of 157 percent in 2005.[1]

Although Wall Street has welcomed these mergers and surging profits of Wellpoint, the insurer has come under increasing scrutiny and fire from state insurance commissioners. At a 2005 hearing in California, for example, Insurance Commissioner John Garamendi called attention to Blue Cross of California's rise in profit margins of 15 percent to 24 percent, together with declines of its MLRs from 80 percent of premiums in 2000 to 68 percent in 2004. What could account for such a drastic drop in the percentage of premiums devoted to paying for health care?

The insurer was accused of cherry-picking. Especially controversial have been the company's fastest growing and most profitable plans that offer low premiums in exchange for high-deductible, limited benefit policies. Its Tonik plan, for example, targets healthy young adults with a deductible of $5,000. Rigorous medical underwriting excludes higher-risk individuals, no maternity benefits are provided, and coverage may be changed or terminated for all covered persons under the plan.[2] The enrollment guidelines for Tonik plans are upfront in rejecting the insurance function of pooling risk—"We believe that the cost of covering someone whose health can be predicted to require costly care should not be subsidized by someone with minimal health care needs."[3]

The regional Vice President for Blue Cross defends these plans by saying that their popularity demonstrates that they are meeting a need, and that "If we were offering a product that people didn't like, they don't have to buy it."[4] That statement reveals how far the nation's largest private insurer has strayed from the original service mission of its Blue Cross predecessor between 1930 and 1950.

Despite growing public outcry over high profit margins, Wellpoint adheres closely to its business plan with a high priority to ease investor concerns. Wall Street maintains an especially close watch on MLRs. When a fourth-quarter 2006 MLR came in at 81.1 percent, down from 81.3 percent in the third quarter but higher than the 2005 level of 79.9 percent, for example, Wellpoint felt compelled to reassure investors that its premium pricing would outpace medical costs. The company noted that its fourth-quarter 2006 net income was up by 23 percent, and that it anticipated that medical costs, which went up by less than 8 percent in 2006, to remain at that level in 2007.

With legislative proposals being promoted in the State Legislature to require insurers to spend at least 85 percent of premium revenue on patient care, Wellpoint CEO Leonard Glasscock worries that such a requirement would limit patient access to affordable benefits, since health plans would be unable to offer certain lower-priced products.[5]

Meanwhile, state regulators in California in mid-2007 were investigating a $950 million dividend payment sent by Blue Cross of California to its Indianapolis-based parent company Wellpoint, a figure almost seven times greater than previous agreements with the State to limit such payments in order to keep premiums affordable and preserve reasonable benefits.[6]

As a result of its strategic mergers, Wellpoint has become the largest processor of claims for Medicare and the leading operator of state Medicaid managed care plans. The insurer announced in 2007 the selection of a new CEO, Angela Braly, an attorney who had served as chief counsel and governmental affairs strategist for the company. The outgoing CEO, Leonard Glasscock had led the company on an eight-year acquisition journey that increased its revenue more than nine-fold to $57 billion in 2006. At a time when Democrats in Congress are planning hearings on public managed care companies, Braly's promotion over other more senior executives could be viewed as a strategy to defend the company's interests in government programs.[7]

United Health Group

Although United Health Group now ranks second behind Wellpoint in membership at about 28 million, it leads the industry in profits, as shown in Table 1.2. The Minneapolis-based company has gone through many stages since United Health Care Corporation was established in 1977. In 1998 it became known as United Health Group, launching "a strategic realignment into independent but strategically linked business segments—United Healthcare, Ovations, Uniprise, Specialized Care Services and Ingenix." Products which have been brought forward by this group since then range from electronic medical ID cards and Web-based data systems to a drug safety monitoring system and high-deductible health plans integrated with health savings accounts.[8]

United Health Group has followed a similar pattern as Wellpoint in pursuing strategic acquisitions and mergers to gain market share, particularly in anticipation of expanded public programs financed by the government. It bought AmeriChoice Corp in 2002, a large Medicaid plan provider. In 2005 it purchased PacifiCare Health Systems Inc., one of the largest purveyors of private Medicare plans with a strong market position as well in Medigap supplemental coverage and Medicare Part D prescription drug plans. It also lobbied hard to secure a deal with AARP to sell its branded Medicare Part D drug benefit plans, gaining more than 5 million enrollees by 2007, more than any other insurer.[9]

A pulmonologist turned corporate executive, Dr. William McGuire, as CEO from 1989 to 2006, presided over a growth spurt for United Health Group over those 17 years. The company's stock multiplied by more than 50-fold during his tenure, but in 2006 he became that year's poster boy for corporate greed. After he built United Health into a leading U.S. insurer and had received almost $2 billion in compensation from the Board of Directors, it was disclosed that well-timed backdated stock option grants to him were illegal and that the head of the company's compensation committee had financial ties to him. Backdating of stock options is a fraudulent practice by which recipients can gain extra profits under the pretense that such options were granted on previous dates when share prices were low.[10] It was soon revealed that McGuire had been given $1.6 billion worth of un-exercised stock options.[11] Figure 2.1 shows the financial gains made by the company and McGuire between 1993 and 2006.[12] In the backdating scandal over stock options which followed, McGuire was forced to resign later that year,[13] and later agreed to forfeit about $418 million to settle claims related to backdated stock options.[14]

The new CEO at United Health, Stephen Hemsley, joined the company in 1997 after 23 years with the accounting firm Arthur Anderson. As president and chief operating officer at United Health, he had received $135 million in compensation from 1997 to 2005, including more than $108 million in stock options. His selection as CEO did not entirely remove a cloud of suspicion over the backdating scandal. The company had commissioned an investigation by an outside law firm Wilmer Cutler Pickering Hale & Dorr. Although its report found it likely that almost 80 percent of stock option grants were backdated, it accepted Hemsley's word that he had little or no role in the practice. [15]

In the aftermath of the backdating scandal, the company took immediate action to reassure employers that their United Health plans were secure. Efforts were also made to convince investors of United Health's stock potential. Its third-quarter 2006 net income had gone up by almost 38 percent, and Hemsley promised continued robust growth

Figure 2.1

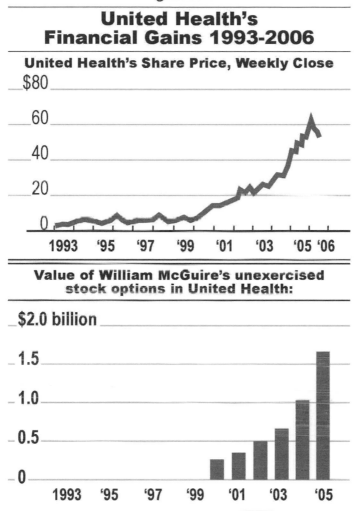

United Health's
Financial Gains 1993-2006

United Health's Share Price, Weekly Close

Source: Thomson Datastream: The Company. Anders G. Rewarding career. As patients, doctors feel pinch, insurer's CEO makes a billion. Wall Street Journal, April 18, 2006: A1.

by stating "We fully intend to continue our current approaches to underwriting and pricing."[16] In October, 2007, United Health reported a 15 percent quarterly profit increase together with a MLR for the previous quarter of 79.5 percent; an "improvement" of 1.6 percent from a year before.[17] Also in 2007, AARP announced seven-year agreements with United Health and Aetna intended to double enrollment in its branded health insurance products while bringing in $1.5 billion in royalty payments to AARP.[18] The conflict of interest of AARP as a membership and advocacy organization will be considered in a later chapter.

At the other end of the age spectrum, health insurance for college and university students has become a growing and lucrative market for private insurers. Such coverage is now strongly suggested by a majority of higher education institutions and required by one third of them. United Health has been quick to exploit this market with extremely low MLRs and high profit margins. At Florida's Palm Beach Community College, for example, its MLR is 42.6 percent for the spring 2008 semester, and has been as low as 10.2 and 13.8 percent in previous semesters (ie., retaining more than 86 percent of premium income for overhead and profits for "coverage" of relatively healthy young people with scanty policies). United Health defends its pricing policies in this way: (we allow school administrators) "to customize plans to meet the needs of their unique student populations. Administrators strive to balance benefits with affordability and act in the best interests of their students."[19]

Aetna

As the third largest U.S. health insurer, Hartford, CT-based Aetna now covers more than 15 million group insurance members. According to its Web site, it provides employer-sponsored health insurance in all 50 states, individual coverage in 17 states, and was the first national full-service health insurer to offer a consumer-directed health plan. The company has had a particularly turbulent experience since the early 1990s, prompting James Robinson, health economist at the University of California Berkeley School of Public Health, to conduct an 18-month case study of the company. His resulting report *From Managed Care to Consumer Health Insurance: The Fall and Rise of Aetna*, documents the company's negative experience with its managed care programs and turnaround to renewed profitability. Having aggressively pursued growth in the managed care sector in the early 1990s, Aetna became the biggest player in the industry by the mid-1990s with 21 million enrollees in capitated managed care plans.[20, 21]

That success was short lived, however, as Aetna soon bore the brunt of a consumer backlash against network restrictions, utilization review, and bad press resulting from denials of care and abandonment of HMO markets. Rebounding from this backlash, Aetna gave up on a mission of growth at all costs, while recommitting itself to profitable growth, with prices outpacing costs. In this transition, Aetna made sharp cutbacks in its managed care plans, withdrawing from Medicare + Choice HMOs in any counties with 65 percent Medicare enrollment and leaving State Medicaid plans altogether. The company emerged from this makeover as a smaller but more profitable multi-product insurer with more emphasis on preferred provider organization (PPO) and health savings account (HSA) products and a new culture of pricing discipline and cost vigilance. Robinson noted the downside of this turnaround, however, in his conclusion of this case study:[22]

> *"The implications of its turnaround are less unambiguously positive for the health system as a whole, however. The employment-based health insurance system is proving to be less willing and able to perform the redistributive functions of social insurance in addition to the risk-spreading functions of market insurance---. Aetna's improved ability to predict and price risk will expose it to obloquy as a failure at social insurance rather than to praise as a success at market insurance. In the health care sector, where no one agrees on the appropriate division of labor between the public and private sectors, no good deed goes unpunished."*

Aetna's new directors soon generated excellent returns to investors. In 2005, it was one of the industry's leading stocks, rising by 51 percent. Such success, however, remains fragile with Wall Street, as other insurers have found. When its MLR rose from 77.9 percent to 79.4 percent from the first quarter of 2005 to that of 2006, its stock fell by 20 percent as investors became concerned about slow growth in enrollment and whether premiums could keep pace with costs of care. [23] Accordingly, Aetna is aggressively marketing new products to younger and healthier enrollees where risks are low and profits higher. Here are two examples of current Aetna products:

- A limited benefit plan with a $250 in-network deductible ($350 out of network), prescription drug card covering a monthly maximum of $35, and a $10,000 maximum benefit cap[24]
- High deductible plans in California with in-network deductibles of $5,000 for individuals and $10,000 for families (double if out-of-network), plus fees beyond Aetna's allowable schedule[25]

Summary

This chapter has demonstrated the sensitivity of Wall Street analysts and investors to profits and medical loss ratios of the largest three health insurers. The Big Three are dependent on investors' expectations that big profits and healthy returns will continue indefinitely. As we saw in Chapter 1, however, the future viability of employer-sponsored health insurance has been called into question in many quarters, and the individual market is relatively small. In their efforts to keep selling insurance that delivers less and less per premium dollar paid, insurers are moving toward high-deductible, limited benefit plans of less value to enrollees. Many of these plans hardly qualify as "insurance," and health care becomes more unaffordable for more of the population every year.

Two big changes are unfolding: Growth in the private market becomes less likely and the new Democrat-controlled Congress is taking aim at assuring a level playing field in public programs without subsidies for private insurers. What do these changes portend for the future of the industry?

The private health insurance industry maintains that its *raison d'etre* is providing people with more efficiency, choice, and value than public programs. We will assess the evidence for and against these claims in the next three chapters. First, we turn to how the industry really works in everyday practice.

References

1. Hoover's Inc. report for Wellpoint, Inc. Accessed February 28, 2007.
2. Girion L. Health plans come under fire. *Los Angeles Times*, December 2, 2005.
3. Blue Cross of California. Tonik plans Benefits Summary List. Thrill-Seeker (T755). Enrollment Guidelines. Accessed January 25, 2007 at http://www.toni-kplans.com/thrill_seeker_CA.pdf.
4. Ibid #2.
5. Brin D.W. Wellpoint's costs rise but 2007 targets stand. *Wall Street Journal*, January 25, 2007: C8.
6. Girion L. Wellpoint dividend is questioned. *Los Angeles Times*, May 26, 2007.
7. Freudenheim M. Top lawyer at Wellpoint is selected as next chief. *New York Times*, February 27, 2007:C3.
8. Web site of United Health Group, accessed February 28, 2007.
9. Zwang J.,& Fuhrmans V. Government pays growing share of health costs. *Wall Street Journal*, February 21, 2007:A1.
10. Bandler J. & Forelle C. Embattled CEO to step down at United Health. *Wall Street Journal*, October 16, 2006:A1.
11. Appleby J. CEO's stock options force restatement at United Health. *USA Today*, May 12, 2006:B8.
12. Anders G. Rewarding career. As patients, doctors feel pinch, insurer's CEO makes a billion. *Wall Street Journal*, April 18, 2006:A1.
13. Bandler J., Forelle C. Bad options. How a giant insurer decided to oust hugely successful CEO. *New York Times*, December 7, 2006:A1.
14. Dash E. Former chief will forfeit $418 million. *New York Times*, December 7, 2007:C1.
15. Dash E. New CEO shadowed by options. *New York Times*, October 17, 2006: C1.
16. Fuhrmans V. United Health on the mend. *Wall Street Journal*, October 20, 2006:B4.
17. Associated Press. United Health posts 15 percent profit increase and raises its full-year forecast. *New York Times*, October 19, 2007:C4.
18. Appleby J., & Wolf R. AARP deals could double its HMO membership. *USA Today*, April 17, 2007:3B.
19. Elgin, B, Silver-Greenberg, J. Is your kid covered? Insurers make big profits from college students, but some families are left with huge bills. Business Week, May 8, 2008
20. Robinson J.C. From managed care to consumer health insurance: The fall and rise of Aetna. *Health Aff (Millwood)* 23(2):43-55, 2004.

21. Lagnado L. Old-line Actna adopts managed care tactics and stirs a backlash. *Wall Street Journal*, July 29, 1998.
22. Ibid #20, 54.
23. Fuhrmans V. Rise in Aetna's medical-cost ratio spooks investors. *Wall Street Journal*, April 28, 2006:A3.
24. Lee K. Second look: High costs and insurer interest are reviving limited benefit medical plan reputation. *Employee Benefit News*, May 2005.
25. Aetna Web site for California. McCanne D. Comment in *Quote of the Day*, December 13, 2005.

CHAPTER 3

From "Cherry Picking" to "Denial Management": How the Industry Really Works

The private health insurance industry holds itself up as providing more efficiency, choice, and value than "one size fits all" public programs. Marketers of private plans tout the advantages of policies tailored to the specific needs of individuals and their families, designed to meet only the benefits they might need at affordable prices. Behind this rhetoric, however, are everyday practices of the industry which call these claims into question.

This chapter has two goals: (1) to examine common practices which limit access, choice, and value of private insurance products, and also which erode the public's trust in the industry; and (2) to briefly consider the implications of these practices for access, equity, and quality of U.S. health care.

Modus Operandi of Private Health Insurance Industry

The methods by which the insurance industry operates to protect its financial interests are varied and, taken collectively, show how committed it is to doing what it takes even at the expense of the patient. They fall into the following four categories, many with several subtypes. We will discuss each in turn:

1. Practices that limit access.
2. Practices restricting choice.
3. Practices limiting value of coverage.
4. Practices that reveal the industry's lack of integrity.

Practices Which Limit Access

As we saw in Chapter 1, being uninsured or underinsured raises serious financial barriers to access to necessary health care for many millions of Americans. Fear of the cost of health care leads many pa-tients to delay or avoid care of both acute and chronic health problems. Many physicians refuse to see patients without adequate insurance. Although limited care can be obtained through emergency rooms, the costs are much higher than care in physicians' offices and followup outpatient care is often not available or affordable. The practice of un-derwriting and re-underwriting based on claims experience allows pri-vate insurers to avoid coverage of enrollees who most need adequate coverage. Here are three typical ways by which private insurers limit their exposure to "medical losses."

1. Outright denial

Health insurance is frequently denied, especially in the indi-vidual market, on the basis of pre-existing conditions, often trivial. Applicants may find themselves uninsurable at any price by what has been called "hangnail underwriting." These typical examples illustrate the point.[1]

- A 39-year old man left his job as a legislative chief of staff with the Los Angeles County Commission on Insurance only to find that he could not obtain health insurance af-ter starting his own marketing and public affairs consult-ing business. Although he was a non-smoker and had never had major surgery, he was rejected by three of California's largest insurers (Blue Cross, Blue Shield, and PacifiCare) on the basis of asthma, among other things. He was finally able to secure coverage through the State's high-risk pool at steep rates.
- A 27-year-old woman in excellent health was denied cover-age because she had seen a psychologist for three months after breaking up with her boyfriend.[2]
- A 46-year-old software consultant in Orem, Utah was denied coverage by American Medical Security, later acquired by California-based PacifiCare. A non-smoker, non-drinker of normal weight, he was turned down because of a history of sinus infections (none in previous six years) and depres-sion well managed on medication.[3]

Insurers are reluctant to disclose their underwriting procedures and denial rates, typically citing privacy rules. However, a new law was passed in California in 2006 requiring insurers to report their un-derwriting guidelines to the State's Department of Insurance and the Department of Managed Care. Table 3.1 lists conditions used by Cali-fornia health insurers in 2006 to deny coverage or raise premiums, according to regulators' postings, rejection letters, and interviews with brokers.[4]

Many insurers impose other categorial reasons to reject appli-cants for health insurance. Three large California insurers (Blue Shield, PacificCare and HealthNet), for example, reject entire categories of

Table 3.1

CONDITIONS USED BY CALIFORNIA INSURERS AS UNDERWRITING GUIDELINES TO DENY COVERAGE, 2006

AIDS	Hepatitis
Allergies	Herpes
Arthritic	High blood pressure
Asthma	Impotence
Attention deficit disorder	Infertility
Autism	Irritable bowel syndrome
Bed-wetting	Joint sprain
Breast implants	Kidney infections
Cancer	Lupus
Cerebral palsy	Mild depression
Chronic bronchitis	Muscular dystrophy
Chronic fatigue syndrome	Migraines
Chronic sinusitis	Miscarriage
Cirrhosis	Pregnancy
Cystitis	"expectant fatherhood"
Diabetes	Planned adoption
Ear infections	Psoriasis
Epilepsy	Recurrent tonsillitis
Gender reassignment	Renal failure
Heart disease	Ringworm
Hemochromatosis (a common	Severe mental disorders
disorder that causes the body to	Sleep apnea
absorb too much iron)	Stroke
	Ulcers and varicose veins

Source: De Moro R.A., Executive Director of California Nurses Association, as cited in http://www.healthcareforall.org/chronicle3. html, February 26, 2007.

workers, such as roofers, pro athletes, dockworkers, police officers, firefighters, and migrant workers. A medical history that involves any of dozens of widely prescribed medications, such as Celebrex, Prevacid, and Allegra, can also result in denial of coverage. The industry responds to criticism by defending its need to avoid high-risk enrollees in order to keep premiums affordable. A spokesperson for Wellpoint, the largest health insurer in the country and the parent company for Blue Cross of California, argues self-servedly that "guaranteed issue can price people out of the market, and as public policy, it achieves the opposite goal of getting more people insured."[5]

The use of genetic conditions by insurance underwriters to screen out potentially risky patients represents an even more ominous threat to the insurability of Americans. The Health Insurance Portability and Accountability Act (HIPAA) of 1996 expressly bans a group health insurance plan from using genetic information to determine eligibility or continued eligibility for coverage. HIPAA further prohibits insurers from treating genetic information as a "pre-existing condition in the absence of the diagnosis of the condition related to such information." Individuals can only be denied if they have symptoms of genetic disease, not because of a genetic marker for the condition. Yet a 2007 national study by researchers at the Johns Hopkins Berman Institute of Bioethics, the Johns Hopkins Bloomberg School of Public Health; the Cleveland Clinic Foundation, the National Institutes of Health, and Georgetown University, found that individuals with genetic conditions were twice as likely to be denied insurance than individuals with other chronic illnesses. More than 60 percent of the 597 study participants believe that health insurers can obtain medical information about them without their permission.[6]

There is good reason for patients to believe that insurers can get medical information on their health status without their permission, as illustrated by recent events in California. For example, Blue Cross of California, the state's largest for-profit insurer, has been sending out letters to physicians asking them to review their patients' applications for health insurance to assess whether any pre-existing conditions have not been disclosed. An accompanying letter to the physicians advised them that Blue Cross has the right to cancel coverage for enrollees who fail to disclose "material medical history", even including "pre-existing pregnancies." In response to an investigative report by the

Los Angeles Times, the president of the California Medical Association recently had this to say:

> *"We're outraged that they are asking doctors to violate the sacred trust of patients to rat them out for medical information that patients would expect their doctors to handle with the utmost secrecy and confidentiality."*[7] *On the following day, Blue Cross of California dropped that review policy with this limp statement: "This letter is no longer necessary and, in fact, was creating a misimpression and causing some members and providers undue concern."* [8]

There are other subtle ways in which insurers can cherry pick their enrollees. These two examples make the point.

- Medicare beneficiaries seeking additional private coverage are frequently asked this question by insurers: "In general, compared to other people your age, would you say your health is excellent, very good, good, fair or poor?" Since there is a five-fold difference in future health costs between the excellent and poor categories, this survey becomes a handy tool for screening out higher-risk patients.[9]
- Many marketing seminars for private Medicare plans have been held on second floors of buildings without elevators or access by wheelchair, effectively creating a barrier to enrollees who, by virtue of mobility problems, would be higher-risk enrollees.[10]

"Denial management" has become a growth industry of its own within the private health insurance industry aimed at denying doctors and hospitals' claims for services provided. An ongoing battle is being waged between insurers and physicians, clinics and hospitals over payment for services. This fight has escalated to the point where about 30 percent of physicians' claims are initially denied. Another wasteful expense in this fight: Each side, providers vs insurance companies, spends about $10 billion a year for denial management services provided by specialized intermediaries. Ingenix, for example, as a unit of United Health Group Inc, the nation's second largest private insurer, markets its products to both sides of the battle, selling insurers systems to screen physicians' claims while selling software systems to physicians that will "help you take a more assertive stance on fair and accurate payment." Another example is Boston-based Athenahealth, a company helping physicians to secure payment for services rendered. Its remarkable growth in the last six years is shown in Figure 3.1.[11]

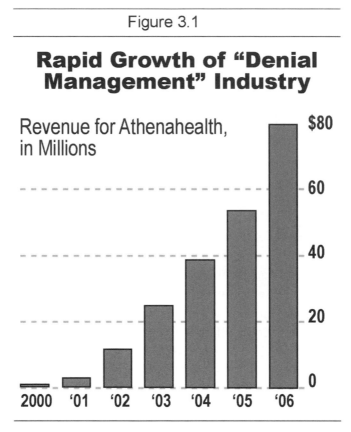

Figure 3.1

Rapid Growth of "Denial Management" Industry

Revenue for Athenahealth, in Millions

2000 '01 '02 '03 '04 '05 '06

Source: The Company. Fuhrmans V. Billing battle. Fights over health claims spawn a new arms race. *Wall Street Journal*, February 14, 2007: A1.

2. Bait and switch

Another common way in which private insurers cherry pick the market is by offering initial premiums at attractive rates to gain market share, than ratcheting up the premiums on annual renewals for those at higher risk for claims. These examples illustrate variations on this theme.

- Insurers often add new restrictions in fine print, such as steep surcharges for top-tier hospitals and new co-payments for cancer radiation treatments, which may render continued coverage unaffordable.[12]
- Since private insurers' coverage policies and rates change frequently from year to year, many insurers are requiring "active enrollment," whereby enrollees are forced to make new selections each year and may find their previous coverage unaffordable and end up in a "default" plan with less coverage.[13]
- Regence BlueShield raised premiums for 137,000 individual-plan enrollees by an average of 19 percent in 2007 (an increase of 40 percent for 16,000 of them); when challenged by Washington Insurance Commissioner Mike Kriedler for bait and switch tactics, a Regence spokesman could only respond "We offer good value to our members."[14]
- Humana jumped early into the Medicare Part D prescription drug benefit market, taking a leading market share by offering low starting premiums; it then re-designed its benefit for 2007 by eliminating brand-name doughnut hole coverage (See Glossary) for patients with higher drug costs and hiking its premiums, even "referring" enrollees to a competitor, Sierra Health Services, without its consent.[15] For the third quarter of 2007, Humana reported record profits of $302 million, mostly gained from its Medicare business, while adding $6.8 million to the retirement account of its CEO, Mike McCallister, who already took in about the same amount in salary.[16] The 2007 premiums for its PDP Standard drug-benefit plan went up by 71 percent over 2005 levels.[17]
- In the first major investigation of Medicare marketing, the Oklahoma Insurance Commissioner received reports from 39 states of complaints about misrepresentations by insurance agents and insurers, including fraudulent practices like falsifying signatures on applications. Humana, which paid its agents $250 for each sale of a Medicare Advantage plan (five times the commission paid for a prescription drug plan), was found to have been involved in widespread mis-

conduct and ordered to take corrective action to protect consumers from high-pressure bait and switch sales tactics. [18]
In some instances, civil and criminal cases have resulted. In
Georgia, for example, state investigators found some agents
who had enrolled dead people using information lifted from
their Medicare records.[19]

3. Cancellation of policies

Although individual enrollees in group insurance plans have
some protection against being dropped from their coverage, insurers
can cancel policies for an entire group or withdraw from the market.
Medicare + Choice (M + C) HMOs did just that in recent years. About
one-third of M + C enrollees across the country lost their coverage
when their plans left their counties for lack of sufficient profitability.[20]
For-profit HMOs owned by large national corporations were more than
twice as likely than not-for-profit HMOs to exit markets. [21]

Insurers employ two common tactics to create loopholes to deny
people coverage in the individual market. One is the application omission game: any time an initial application has an omission, intended
or not, a policy can be canceled. Second, many applications for health
insurance contain questions that are either vague or confusing. When
insurers want to cancel coverage, answers to these confusing questions
can then form the basis to question adequate disclosure, giving them
their loophole.

Two examples show how this worked in individual cases.

- A Los Angeles woman lost her Blue Cross coverage after a
  routine physician's visit; the reason given for her canceled
  coverage was her failure to report a corrective surgery 20
  years earlier. The lack of reporting was no fault of the patient: the application had only asked for a 10-year medical
  history.[22]
- A college student with Blue Shield coverage was hospitalized for gastroenteritis and dehydration, running up a hospital bill of $9,000; the insurer canceled his coverage stating
  that his initial application had omitted mention of past bouts
  of diarrhea, which the student felt were too insignificant to
  report.[23]

These are not isolated cases, but common practices of insurers which have attracted scrutiny by regulators and litigation. In California, the state regulator of HMOs in 2007 fined Blue Cross $1 million for canceling coverage of enrollees for such reasons as becoming pregnant.[24] Blue Cross of California, now owned by Wellpoint, the country's largest health insurer, in 2006 agreed to settle more than 70 lawsuits and claims filed by patients against their canceled policies.[25]

Health Net, another large California insurer with almost 240,000 enrollees in Medicare Advantage plans, was recently fined $1 million by the California Department of Managed Health Care for setting monthly targets for cancellation of policies tied to staff bonuses. One senior analyst received $20,000 in bonuses for cancelling 1,600 policies between 2000 and 2006, saving the company $35.5 million in medical expenses.[26] To cite another example, Las Vegas-based Sierra Health terminated drug coverage for 2,300 HIV-positive Medicare Advantage enrollees, improperly claiming that they had not paid their plan premiums.[27]

Practices Restricting Choice

Despite their repeated claims of providing increased choice to patients, private health plans much more often restrict enrollees' choices. These restrictions come in many forms, including misleading and devious marketing, changes of in-network providers and hospitals, withdrawal of plans from the area, and lock in rules preventing enrollees from making changes they desire.

Volatile change of plan policies is more the rule than the exception. A 2003 study found typical annual turnover rates of patients' insurance coverage of 20 percent, often requiring change of physicians.[28] Private Medicare + Choice HMOs dropped about one-third of enrollees as they withdrew from the market between 1999 and 2003 when their subsidized payments fell below their financial goals. [29] Even after a $1 billion infusion of Medicare reimbursement in 2001, few such programs re-entered the market.[30] A 2004 study found that only one-half of disenrolled patients were able to keep their primary care physicians.[31] Each of these instances above shows the allegiance of insurers to their profits, not to their enrollees, an allegiance that, in other countries with single payer insurance, does not exist. This is a point to which we will return later.

Here are three examples, across the country, of how health plans limit choices of both patients and physicians while disrupting continuity of care.

- In 2006, Oxford Health Plans, a subsidiary of United Health Group, told hundreds of physicians and thousands of its enrollees that it would no longer pay for medical care at Jamaica Hospital Medical Center in Queens, New York. They were given one month to make alternative arrangements. In addition, some physicians were advised that they would no longer be permitted to participate in the Oxford plans, while many patients were told to find other physicians. Jamaica Hospital has chronic financial difficulties and serves a largely poor population with many immigrants and uninsured people. Conflicts between the hospital and Oxford had begun when the insurer failed to increase payments to the hospital as agreed upon in a new contract in 2004. Jamaica incurred losses of tens of millions of dollars, and brought suit against the insurer in 2006. Meanwhile, continuity of care was disrupted for large numbers of patients.[32]
- In 2006, the San Diego-based Sharp physician network imposed this ultimatum on its physicians—all your senior patients must enroll in one health plan, Secure Horizons, within the next three months or you can no longer use Sharp's services in San Diego County. Forty-five physicians had only a few days to accept or reject this ultimatum. If they decided to work only with Sharp, their non-Secure Horizons patients would have to switch to that insurer or change to other participating primary care physicians. More than 20,000 patients were affected by this ultimatum. Neighboring community hospitals stood to lose patients if more physicians agreed to stay with Sharp, as did those physicians who elected to break from the Sharp network.[33]
- In 2007, United Health Group threatened to fine physicians $50 if any of their patients had laboratory tests done by any laboratory other than Laboratory Corp. of America or other facilities selected by the insurer. Physicians with patients seeking out-of-network services would also be subject

to lower reimbursement or exclusion from United's net-work.[34]

Practices Limiting Value of Coverage

The private health insurance industry is increasingly bringing to market a wide selection of plans of very limited value, marketed aggressively as plans tailored to the needs of individuals and their families. Behind this rhetoric are many policies giving little security against major illness or accident, and hardly qualifying for the word "insurance." The motivation is clear: medical loss ratios are low, thus pleasing investors.

Here are some examples of this growing trend, mostly offered by insurers and employers under the banner of "consumer-directed health care." The term sounds warm and customer-friendly, but it is classic public relations designed to hide the opposite—health insurance that is intended to restrict consumer choice.

1. Limited benefit ("Mini Med") policies (LBPs)

These are targeted to younger, healthier people by such insurers as Aetna, Cigna and AllState. An increasing number of employers are offering LBPs to their workers, especially if they are entry or part-time workers. These plans typically cover some routine and preventive services with low co-payments, but many policies also have low annual caps. They provide little or no coverage for such major needs as surgery or hospitalization. Here are examples of various LBPs now on the market.

- AllState sells a basic cancer policy, starting at $420 a year for family coverage, which pays a one-time benefit of $2,000 if diagnosed for the first time with cancer (other than skin cancer)[35]
- LBPs offered to employees and family members by such large employers as Wall Mart Stores, Inc., McDonald's Corp., and Lowe's, often have annual caps as low as $1,000 to $2,500.[36]
- Aetna Affordable Health Choices caps hospital benefits at $2,000 and accident/ER benefits at $1,000[37]

- Anthem, now part of WellPoint, is marketing its Blue Access Economy Plan with $1,000 deductible which covers three annual physician visits at a $30 co-pay each and a generic drug plan capped at $500[38] ; Anthem's latest entry into the market is its Blue Access Hospital Surgical PPO providing "catastrophic" coverage for most surgeries and hospitalizations, but with deductibles of $1,000 to $5,000 for individual coverage and $3,000 to $15,000 for family coverage[39]
- Mutual of Omaha offers a $25,000 critical-illness policy covering Alzheimer's, blindness or organ transplant at $375 to $400 a year for a 40-year-old man[40]

There are hitches to all of these policies that protect insurers against significant losses and assure them lucrative returns. For example, applicants for critical-illness policies are frequently denied if they already have a covered illness or if several direct relatives have had one. Most of these policies are marketed to people in their 30s and 40s, and new policies are not usually issued after ages 59 or 65.[41]

2. Mental health "carve-outs"

These are subcontracts by insurers to for-profit "behavioral health companies" which separate mental health benefits from other parts of coverage. They get around laws on mental health parity (See Glossary) and deliver the least amount of care for maximal financial return. That is accomplished by imposing barriers to access, including limits on the number of visits to a psychiatrist, the amount of time per visit (eg., 20 minutes), and forcing early discharge from hospitals without arrangements for adequate follow-up care.[42]

3. High-deductible health insurance plans (HDHI), with health savings accounts (HSAs)

The offering of these plans by insurers as part of "consumer directed" health care (CDHC) has led to new layers of expensive but lucrative health care bureaucracy which limits value of coverage. Insurers and investment firms compete for an estimated $1 billion in fees for managing health savings accounts (HSAs); Blue Cross and UnitedHealth have already chartered their own banks for this purpose.[43]

A recent study by investigators at Harvard Medical School has found that many people, especially women and those in their middle years, will be financial losers in these plans. Young women are especially at risk for high out-of-pocket costs, with median expenditures three times higher than for men in the same age group.[44] In addition, some HDHI plans with HSAs cost even more than other HDHI plans not HSA eligible.[45]

4. Medigap plans

Many seniors purchase supplemental health insurance plans (Medigap) to cover some expenses not covered by traditional Medicare. Indeed, health insurance premiums represent the largest health care costs for seniors (8 percent of total expenditures), exceeding the costs of prescription drugs (6 percent), health services (4 percent), and medical supplies (1 percent).[46] However, the actual value of Medigap plans to seniors is open to question. Since Medicare allows payments that are usually much lower than billed charges, the amounts of claims payments for which insurers are obligated are often relatively small. While insurers cover only modest coinsurance and deductibles, their profit margin can be high. As an example, the Senior Classic F Medigap plan of Blue Cross of California in 2001 had a medical-loss ratio of only 62 percent (ie., Blue Cross retained 38 percent of premium income, an especially attractive return for the company and its investors).[47]

5. Medicare Advantage

Proponents of private Medicare plans (HMO, PPO, or private fee-for-service (PFFS) plans, claim that these plans provide added value in benefits for their enrollees compared to traditional Medicare. However, there is scant evidence that this "added value" is worth the government's high overpayments (112 percent average for HMO-PPOs and 119 percent for PFFs). The Centers for Medicare & Medicaid Services (CMS) have no way to monitor the extent of added benefits. CMS is even barred by law from tracking benefits of the most expensive plans, PFFS, to see to what extent these subsidies result in expanded benefits. CMS's Abby Block, who directs the Center for Beneficiary Choices, has acknowledged this loophole in testimony before the House Ways and Means Committee. The costs of this loophole are clear: A PFFS plan can therefore take in an extra $1,000 in annual subsidies while providing enrollees with just one dental cleaning worth $100.[48]

Taken together, these examples show how distant private health insurance is from the paradigm of free market economics. In economic theory, the customer rules supreme, able to demand and receive increasing quality in service at a declining price, threatening to go elsewhere if a company can't deliver. But with health insurance we see the opposite: decreasing service, increasing price, in a context where consumers cannot call the shots. The trend suggested above plays out in only one direction—with increasing benefit to the insurance companies—because their ability to set the rules in their favor vastly outstrips the political power consumers have been able to muster.

Practices Which Reveal the Industry's Lack of Integrity

In addition to the above practices of private insurers which limit access, choice, and value of their products, the industry has many other standard practices that are dishonest and unfair. Any one instance by itself can be seen as just one more egregious practice. But collectively, they show just what private health insurance is really about, and why it cannot be easily fixed with a few regulations. These practices take several forms.

1. Inadequate Disclosure

Many applicants for private health insurance find the details of their coverage to be incomprehensible and buried in fine print beyond their understanding. Even when private plans take steps to provide accurate information to applicants, these efforts often fall short of their needs. For example, a recent report by the Medicare Rights Center and California Health Advocates found that call centers established by Part D prescription drug plans frequently fail to provide the information seniors need to make appropriate enrollment decisions.[49] Many insurers also fail to notify enrollees of changes in their coverage. There are more than 50 Part D drug plans in every state except Alaska and Hawaii, yet United Health Group, one of the largest of the plans, had not sent out notices of changes for 200,000 of its enrollees by the required deadline in 2006.[50]

2. Inappropriate Disclosure

Privacy breaches of personal health records by private insurers are not at all uncommon. As an example, the Government Accountability Office (GAO) found that 90 percent of private Medicare plans outsourced some services to contractors in 2005, and that nearly one-half of the contractors had privacy breaches within the previous two years. Unlike Medicare itself, Medicare Advantage contractors are not required to report breaches of privacy. [51]

3. Deceptive Marketing

We have already seen some examples of misrepresentations by insurance agents and insurers in our foregoing discussion of bait and switch marketing. But the range of deceptive marketing practices is indeed broad, and these practices are widespread. For example, case-workers at the Medicare Rights Center in New York have received these kinds of reports from dual-eligibles (people meeting eligibility for both Medicare and Medicaid) in New York State:

- brokers coming unsolicited to their doors and posing as government Medicare representatives;
- brokers offering $200 drugstore coupons for signing up with a plan;
- brokers telling people with Medicare that they "must" sign up for their plan by a certain date or else they will be fined by Medicare;
- brokers telling dual eligibles that they will lose their Medicaid or Medicare coverage if they do not sign up for that particular plan;
- brokers going door-to-door in senior homes after they were invited to one of the apartments;
- plan representatives setting up in the lobbies of senior centers with their marketing materials, ready to process enrollments and give presentations;
- brokers fooling dual eligibles at a senior center into signing up for a Medicare Advantage plan by telling them they were signing up for a raffle to win prizes;
- insurance brokers working for Health First telling dual eligibles that they needed three cards to receive medical services: their Medicare, Medicaid and Health First cards;

- brokers misrepresenting the coverage offered by downplaying formulary restrictions and doctors' networks, or telling people with Medicare that they will not need referrals to see specialists (when they will);
- brokers giving potential enrollees false information about their doctors being part of the plan's network (the enrollees are subsequently billed large sums of money when they continue to see their doctors who are actually out of network);
- plans advertising services already covered under Medicare/ Medicaid as uniquely covered under MA plans (such as dental and transportation coverage);
- brokers presenting appeals processes as very easy to navigate and taking very little time.

These problems are most common with brokers working for WellCare, Health First, and Touchstone.[52] Here are two illustrations of how these practices adversely impact patients at both ends of the country, from the records of the Medicare Rights Center and California Health Advocates.

- Mr. And Mrs. W., who live near Buffalo, New York, joined Blue Cross/Blue Shield's Senior Blue plan late last year. In February, Mr. W. called MRC because none of his wife's doctors participated in the plan's provider network. A plan salesman neglected to mention that the couple would not be able to choose any doctor they wished to see, which was what they were used to under Original Medicare. A plan representative told Mr. W. that his wife could not go to her regular doctors. The couple wants to drop the plan and return to Original Medicare. But it is too late. No changes could be made after March 31 until the next year.[53]
- In California, Ms. R., a conservator for a person with Medicare who lives in assisted living, reported that an agent came to her door in late December 2006, uninvited, after driving up and down her block. He had a clipboard in hand that had a list of names, one of which was her client's, with Ms. R.'s address as a contact. The agent began to ask if her client,

who was enrolled in a particular sponsor's PDP product, was aware of the same sponsor's PFFS plan and the current limited Open Enrollment Period then in effect. He extolled the "improved program with more benefits" for current enrollees in the PDP plan. He opened a folder and showed the "improved" eye care and hearing aid care benefits and personal items allowed each month under the PFFS plan. He told her any doctor could bill the plan instead of Medicare, and, "you can choose your own doctor." She was then told that she needed to make a decision by the end of the month, and he would have to pick up the application after she filled it out and "signed here." He asked her to call him when she had completed it so that he could pick it up. The agent told her he had talked to 39 clients, and 36 of them had already signed up.[54]

In June 2007, a month after a Senate committee heard testimony about these abuses, seven U.S. insurers, including United Health Group and Humana, suspended marketing of the most lucrative private Medicare plan, PFFS, which receives overpayments 19 percent above the costs of traditional Medicare.[55] It is not surprising that this decision came at a time when Congress was considering cutting back on these overpayments, and when the Medicare Payment Advisory Commission (MEDPAC) had just reported that PFFS plans had used less than one-half of their overpayments to provide additional benefits.[56]

4. Hidden Conflicts of Interest

Conflicts of interest (COIs) abound in the marketing process of private health insurance products, about which many purchasers have little or no awareness. These examples show how concealed these COIs can be.

- As an employee-benefits consultant for the Columbus (Ohio) Public School District in 2001, Kevin Grady was paid $35,000 a year to help the District select a health insurer. On Grady's recommendation, the District switched its health insurance to United Health Group Inc., only to find several years later that he had received $547,138 from the company for helping it to secure the District's business. The Ohio District of Insurance ordered that $137,000 be paid in restitution to the District and United Health agreed to pay a $125,000 penalty to settle the matter without admitting wrongdoing.[57]

- EHealthInsurance is a Sunnyvale, California company established in 1997 for more efficient marketing of health insurance to individuals. It has developed partnerships with 135 insurers, including Aetna and Cigna. When policies are sold, EHealthInsurance takes an average 20 percent cut of the annual premium charged by the insurer, and also receives about 10 percent of premium costs for future renewals, even when not renewed through its own Web site.[58]

- Some insurers set up non-profit associations as false fronts to attract individual enrollees to their for-profit plans without disclosure of their links to the purchaser. Many states exempt these associations from regulations, especially concerning rate increases, because of their "not-for-profit" status. Golden Rule Financial Group, one of the leading providers of association policies, was bought by United Health Group Inc. in 2003. According to a 2004 report by Families USA, these loose associations, which require purchasers to join and pay dues to the association, are often under the operational and financial control of insurers.[59]

- Ohio-based Aon Corporation markets Sterling PFFS Medicare plans, as do Humana and United HealthGroup. As we have seen earlier, PFFS plans receive the highest overpayments from the government compared to traditional Medicare (119 percent), are virtually unregulated, and can market their plans year-round. These advantages were quietly tucked into legislation by then-House Speaker Dennis Hastert (R, IL), who had received almost $20,000 from Aon Corporation for his 2006 campaign.[60]

Beyond the marketing area, hidden conflicts of interest lurk beyond our awareness elsewhere in the industry. A recent example concerns the process used by the industry to calculate reimbursement rates for physicians. UnitedHealth Group, the nation's second largest private insurer, owns Ingenix, a little-known company that collects and compiles billing information from UnitedHealth and other insurers. This database is then used to determine out-of-network reimbursement rates for physicians' services. The American Medical Association has had a long-standing lawsuit filed against Ingenix and various United-Health companies, alleging that the data are manipulated and adjusted downward in an unfair way. The conflict of interest is obvious. Insurers stand to gain financially if they can pay less for medical services and lower their medical loss ratios.[61]

5. Devious Dealings with Physicians

It has been well documented that more than 450 health insurance plans across the country use software programs produced by McKesson Corporation of San Francisco to automatically reduce reimbursement to physicians by changing standard billing codes.[62] Recent years have seen a running battle between U.S. physicians and private health insurers over reimbursement and billing practices. That battle has escalated to litigation, even to the point of invoking the federal Racketeer Influenced and Corrupt Organizations (RICO) Act in a class-action lawsuit. That suit was upheld by a federal appeals court in 2004. At that time the judge described the case as involving "almost all doctors versus almost all major health maintenance organizations." Table 3.2 lists the physicians' allegations in the lawsuit.[63] As a result of this and similar litigation, insurers have been forced to agree to large settlements, including Cigna ($540 million)[64] and most recently 23 Blue Cross and Blue Shield companies which together cover 50 million enrollees.[65] In addition to cash settlements, insurers typically agree to provide more transparency in physician reimbursement and review procedures.

Despite these settlements, physicians continue to be frustrated and burdened by added bureaucracy in dealing with private insurers. They must still employ additional administrative staff to track their billings, which often fall short of correctly billed charges. As an example, Pediatric Alliance, which includes pediatricians in a dozen offices in and around Pittsburgh, spends more than $250,000 each year for salaries of eight billing clerks who track payments owed by insurers and patients.[66] At the other end of the age spectrum, a 2007 national survey by the AMA found that more than one-half of physicians reported that their payments from private Medicare Advantage plans were below

---

Table 3.2

Allegations in the Class-Action Lawsuit by Physicians against Insurers.

All insurers
Denying valid claims
Deliberately delaying claims
Using undisclosed cost-based criteria to assess the medical necessity
  of claims
Providing monetary incentives to claims reviewers to deny or delay payments
Implementing claims-processing software to adjust automatically (by
  "downcoding" or "bundling") or deny claims without notice
Using overwhelming market power to coerce physicians to accept
  billing practices
Failing to provide a reasonable appeals process for claims

In capitation schemes
Retaining or adjusting capitation payments illegally
Reimbursing physicians when patients initially enroll rather than waiting until
  enrollees need services
Failing to pass along savings from pharmaceutical rebates or pharmaceutical
  and hospital-use risk pools to physicians who share in costs and risks

Source; Kesselheim A.S., & Brennan T.A. Overbilling vs. downcoding-The
battle between physicians and insurers. N Engl J Med 352(9):855-7, 2005.

---

those of traditional Medicare and that 45 percent of their patients in Medicare Advantage PFFS plans had encountered denial of services generally covered by Original Medicare. [67]

One core claim of private health insurance is that, because it is driven by the profit motive, it is more efficient than a government program could ever be. One easy place to test this is in claims processing. If this was true, claims processed by the hyper efficient private sector should be vastly faster and better than the public sector. Yet, a 2006 report from AthenaHealth, a major claims processing company serving both sides of the conflict between insurers and physicians, found that the most reliable organization for paying physician charges in full when first submitted (92 percent of the time) was Medicare. In contrast, Wellpoint, the nation's largest private insurer, which should have enormous advantages over other insurers by virtue of its economies of scale, trailed behind Medicare, paying physician charges in full when first submitted just 86.3 percent of the time.[68]

6. Profiteering Through Insider Stock Sales

WellCare is a big player in private Medicare and Medicaid plans. It went public in 2004 with an IPO stock price of $17.00. Since then its stock has outperformed Standard & Poor's 500-stock index by 428 percent. As its stock prices surged, a number of its executives and directors sold their shares with little regard for restrictions on insider sales. More than $47 million worth of stock was sold in 2007 before the company's headquarters was raided by the FBI and other federal and state agencies in October of that year. Its stock price fell $72.50 on news of the raid (by 63 percent), with a $3 billion decline in its market capitalization as the investigation proceeded. [69]

7. Outright Fraud

Fraud has been an ongoing problem within the private health insurance industry for many years. Between 1993 and 2002, the federal government recovered more than $400 million in settlements from insurers making false claims.[70] As fiscal intermediaries for Medicare, Blue Cross/Blue Shield plans have been successfully prosecuted by the government for such practices as falsification of audits, administrative costs, and number of claims processed.[71] A 2004 GAO report found widespread insurance scams in every state involving more than 15,000 employers and 200,000 policyholders. [72]

A 2006 report by the *Kansas City Star* concluded that misconduct and fraud among insurance agents is widespread and getting worse. Common abuses include selling unlicensed products or unsuitable coverage and stealing purchasers' premiums by failing to forward them to the insurer.[73] Dr. Don McCanne, Senior Health Policy Fellow for Physicians for a National Health Program (PNHP) offers this observation:[74]

> *"Insurance agents have a difficult task. They must help their clients purchase plans that are affordable, that provide adequate financial protection, that will cover preexisting disorders, that will ensure that providers are accessible, and they must be certain that the insurer is reliable and capable of as-*

suming risk. Truth told, there are no health insurance products
that meet all of these standards. So the agent is in a position
of assisting his/her client in selecting a compromised product,
and may not even be able to provide any product if costs are
prohibitive or medical underwriting prevents coverage."

What are the Implications of These Practices
for U.S. Health Care?

The foregoing has documented that the problems of the private
health insurance industry are systemic. They are widespread and involve the nation's largest insurers, not just "a few bad apples." This
is understandable from a business perspective. We have a financing
system filled with perverse incentives, and the financial rewards for
insurers and their investors are enormous. In a competitive for-profit
industry, insurers risk losing market share unless they pursue the kinds
of practices described here. Losers in this struggle are likely to be swal-
lowed up in the consolidation dance described earlier.

Since cost containment of escalating health care costs is nowhere
on the horizon, U.S. health care is in crisis. In order to keep their industry afloat, private insurers are offering less valuable "coverage" to
a declining employer-based and individual market, while expanding
their markets in public programs through still generous government
subsidies. There is great irony in this, as we saw in the opening chapter, since the private insurance industry continues to claim its greater
efficiency and value than public programs, and since private insurers
blatantly shift sicker people into public safety net programs by avoiding coverage of sicker people.

As currently configured, private health insurance is designed to
drive costs ever higher. Private insurers are fighting for the right to be
increasingly inefficient by keeping their medical loss ratios (MLRs)
below 80 percent if possible. The standard pro-business argument is
that economies of scale reduce overhead and that the profit motive provides incentives for business to deliver services more efficiently than
the government can do. By these arguments, insurer MLRs should be
rising, not falling. The higher they get the more efficient they should
be, and the lower their overhead should be. Instead, however, large
private insurers use their savings provided by scale to reduce what they

deliver to patients—and fatten the wallets of investors.

This situation is untenable and cannot last. A tipping point is coming. A public and legislative backlash is building against over-payment subsidies in Medicare. America's Health Insurance Plans (AHIP), as the trade group for the industry, has neither incentive nor regulatory ability to rid the industry of misconduct. Further, fragmen-tation of the risk pool by expanding products of less value to healthier people negates the whole point of insurance to share risk widely.

Health care is not just another commodity on the open market. There is a universal need for our population to gain affordable access to necessary health care and to have economic security from the rav-ages of disease and injury without facing bankruptcy for themselves and their families. Lower-income and middle-class Americans, even if insured and employed, are finding access to affordable health care increasingly difficult. As more costs are shifted to patients and their families, people often forgo necessary health care. There can be no quality of health care if it is not accessible, and our health care "sys-tem" is becoming increasingly tiered and inequitable.

It is becoming more obvious every day that major system reform will be required—and soon. Whether the private insurance industry can contribute to needed reforms has become a serious question. The industry is on an unsustainable path and we need to question its future role as a financing mechanism for U.S. health care. Before returning to these questions, however, we need to examine in the next chapter the many myths perpetuated by stakeholders in the present market-based system about health care and health insurance.

References

1. Girion L. Healthy ? Insurers don't buy it: Minor ailments can thwart applicants for individual policies. *Los Angeles Times*, December 31, 2006.
2. Ibid #1.
3. Lueck S. Health concerns. Seeking insurance, individuals face many obstacles. *Wall Street Journal*, May 31, 2005: A1.
4. Ibid #1.

5. Girion L. Health insurers deny policies in some jobs. Common medications also can be deemed too risky in California. *Los Angeles Times*, January 8, 2007.

6. Kass N. E., Medley A. M., Natowicz M.R., Hull S.C., Fallen R.R., et al. Access to health insurance: Experiences and attitudes of those with genetic versus non-genetic medical conditions. *Am J Med Genet* Part A, 143:707-17, 2007.

7. Girion L. Doctors balk at request for data. *Los Angeles Times*, February 12, 2008.

8. Griffith D. Blue Cross drops review policy. *Sacramento Bee*, February 13, 2008:B1.

9. Bierman A.S., Bubolz T.A., Fisher E.S. & Wasson J. H. How well does a single question about health predict the financial health of Medicare managed care plans? *Eff Clin Pract* 2(2) 56, 1999.

10. Neuman P., Maibach E., Dusenbury K., Kitchman M., & Zupp R. Market HMOs to Medicare beneficiaries. *Health Aff (Millwood)* 17(4):132-9, 1998.

11. Fuhrmans V. Billing battle. Fights over health claims spawn a new arms race. *Wall Street Journal*, February 14, 2007: A1.

12. Court J. Insurance: You pay, they bait and switch. *Los Angeles Times*, 2002.

13. Kristof K. M. Big changes for health plans. *Los Angeles Times*, October 9, 2005.

14. Song K.M. Gulp! Regence rate boost averages 19 percent for individual plans. *The Seattle Times*, May 16, 2007.

15. Young J. Feds probe Humana over Rx drug patients. *The Hill*, March 8, 2007.

16. Medicare Rights Center. Who is Medicare for? *Asclepios* 7(43):November 1, 2007.

17. Zhang J. Seniors weigh new options on drug benefit. *Wall Street Journal*, November 13, 2007:D1.

18. Pear R. Insurer faces reprimand in Medicare marketing case. *New York Times*, May 15, 2007:A14.

19. Williamson E. & Lee C. Medicare hard-sell. Abusive tactics found in sales tactics. *Washington Post National Weekly Edition*, May 21-27, 2007, p 24.

20. CMS Medicare Fact Sheet. Centers for Medicare and Medicaid Services, September 2002.

21. Lake T. & Brown R. Medicare + Choice Withdrawals: Understanding Key Factors. Menlo Park, Calif: Kaiser Family Foundation, June 2002.

22. Chan G. State fines Blue Cross $200,000. *Sacramento Bee*, September 22, 2006.

23. Girion L. Blue Shield sued over revoked insurance. *Los Angeles Times*, February 16, 2007.

24. Editorial. Coverage for all. *Sacramento Bee*, March 25, 2007.

25. Girion L. The nation. Blue Cross settling patients' lawsuits. The big insurer, accused of illegally canceling some policies, agrees to pay its ex-customers. *Los Angeles Times*, October 18, 2006;A1.

26. Medicare Rights Center. California-based insurance plan fined $1 million. New York: *Medicare Watch* 10(24):November 27, 2007.

27. Medicare Rights Center. CMS releases MA audit results. *Medicare Watch* 21, October 16, 2007, 35.

28. Franks P., Cameron C., Bertakis K.D. On being new to an insurance plan: health care use associated with the first years in a health plan. *Ann Fam Med* 1:156-61, 2003.

29. Bodenheimer T. The dismal failure of Medicare privatization. Senior Action Network. San Francisco, California, June 2003, p 1.

30. Waldholz M. Prescriptions: Medicare seniors face confusion as HMOs bail out of program. *The Wall Street Journal*, Oct. 3, 2002, p D4.

31. Chernew M.E., Wodchis W.P., Scanlon D.P. & McLaughlin C.G. Overlap in HMO physician networks. *Health Aff (Millwood)* 23(2):91-101, 2004.

32. Perez-Pena R. Insurer-hospital dispute rattles patients in Queens. *New York Times*, May 30, 2006:A19.

33. Clark C. Doctors object to ultimatum on health care. *The San Diego Union-Tribune*, February 26, 2006.

34. Agovino T. Doctors fear new UnitedHealth policy. *Houston Chronicle*, February 14, 2007.

35. McQueen M.P. The shifting calculus of workplace benefits. *Wall Street Journal*, January 16, 2007: D1.

36. Terhune C. Thin cushion. Fast-growing health plan has a catch, $1,000-a-year cap. *Wall Street Journal*, May 14, 2003:A1.

37. Fuhrmans V. More employers try limited health plans. *Wall Street Journal*, January 17, 2006:D1.

38. Fuhrmans V. Health insurers' new target. *Wall Street Journal*, May 31, 2005: B1.

39. Kaiser Daily Health Policy Report. Anthem Blue Cross and Blue Shield to offer limited-benefit plan to employers in five states. November 30, 2007.

40. Silverman E. Getting paid for getting sick. *Wall Street Journal*, July 14, 2005: D1.

41. Ibid #38.

42. Munoz R. Parity or parody. How health care insurers avoid treating mental illness. *The San Diego Union-Tribune*, May 22, 2006.

43. Becker C. One question: credit or debit? As health savings accounts gain in popularity, insurers and the financial services industry want to bank the cash. *Mod Healthcare* 36:6-16, 2006.

44. Woolhandler S. & Himmelstein D.U. Consumer directed healthcare: Except for the healthy and wealthy, it's unwise. *J Gen Intern Med* 22(6):879-81, 2007.

45. Rubenstein S. A hitch on health insurance. Plans that mesh with tax-saving device often cost more. *Wall Street Journal*, June 10-11, 2006:B4.

46. Butrica B.A., Goldwin J.H., & Johnson R.W. Understanding expenditure patterns in retirement. The Urban Institute, January 2005.

47. McCanne D. Comment on reference #42 in "Quote of the Day," February 14, 2005 (don@mccanne.org).

48. Medicare Rights Center. Medicare private plan overpayments: No bang for the buck. *Asclepios* 7(21), May 24, 2007.

49. Press report. Medicare private drug plans fail to offer accurate information to consumers. New York: Medicare Rights Center. October 12, 2006. Full report available at http://www.cahealthadvocates.org/advocacy/2006/10.html.

50. Pear R. Drug plan companies failed to tell of changes. *New York Times,* December 27, 2006:A18.

51. GAO finds widespread privacy breaches of MA plans. *Medicare Watch* 9(1), September 12, 2006.

52. Lipschutz D., Precht F., & Burns B. After the Goldrush: The Marketing of Medicare Advantage and Part D Plans. California Health Advocates and Medicare Rights Center. Issue Brief #4, January 2007, p 10.

53. Ibid #52, p 8.

54. Medicare Rights Center. Too good to be true: The fine print in Medicare private health plan benefits. New York, April 2007, p 8.

55. Bloomberg News. Insurers suspend the marketing of some Medicare plans. *New York Times*, June 16, 2007:B2.

56. Medicare Rights Center. Congress eyes payments to Medicare private plans. *Medicare Watch* 10(5): March 6, 2007.

57. Martinez B. Double bypass. Health-care consultants reap fees from those they evaluate. *Wall Street Journal*, September 18, 2006:A1.

58. Tep R. Click here for coverage. Forbes. com, November 21, 2006.

59. Terhune C. Report raps association insurance. *Wall Street Journal*, March 11, 2004:D3.

60. Medicare Rights Center. Stop this scam. *Asclepios* 7(5):February 1, 2007.

61. Editorial. A rip-off by health insurers? *New York Times*, February 18, 2007.

62. Martinez B. CIGNA to settle suit over cuts in doctor bills. *The Wall Street Journal*, Nov. 27, 2002, p A3.

63. Kesselheim A.S., & Brennan T.A. Overbilling vs. downcoding-The battle between physicians and insurers. *N Engl J Med* 352(9):855-7, 2005.

64. Physicians Financial News. Judge approves $540 million Cigna settlement. March 15, 2004.

65. Fuhrmans V. Health insurers settle dispute on pay with 900,000 doctors. *Wall Street Journal*, April 28, 2007:A3.

66. Freudenheim M. The check is not in the mail. Late payment of medical claims adds to the cost of health care. *New York Times*, May 25, 2006:C1.

67. AMA. American Medical Association calls for financial neutrality in Medicare Advantage. Chicago, IL: May 22, 2007.

68. Ibid #65.

69. Frincus T., & Martinez B. WellCare insider sales mount. *Wall Street Journal*, October 26, 2007:A12.

70. McGinley L. General American to pay $76 million in Medicare case. *The Wall Street Journal*, June 26, 2002, p A2.

71. Sparrow M.K. *License to steal: How fraud bleeds America's health care system*. Boulder, CO: Westview Press, 2000, pp 74-5.

72. Pear R. Inquiry finds sharp increase in health insurance scams. *New York Times*, March 3, 2004, p A12.

73. Morris M. Only wreckage remains when insurance agents breach trust. You think you're covered? You might be surprised, and at the worst possible time. *The Kansas City Star*, December 11, 2006.

74. McCanne D. Quote of the Day (don@mccanne.org, December 12,2006; commenting on reference #75.)

CHAPTER 4

Myths and Mirrors:
How the Industry Perpetuates Itself

*"A lie gets half-way around the world
before the truth gets its pants on."*
—Mark Twain

The above saying of Mark Twain's seems hand crafted for the health insurance industry. A divisive public debate has been waged in this country for at least 75 years over the role of markets and government in health care. Much of this debate has been based on rhetoric, myths, and mirrors which serve the industry well but confuse and distort the issues.

As an example, the Dallas-based National Center for Policy Analysis (NCPA), a conservative think tank, put out an extensive document in 2002 entitled *Twenty Myths about Single-Payer Health Insurance: International Evidence on the Effects of National Health Insurance in Countries Around the World.*[1] This was intended to discredit single-payer national health insurance as a policy option for the U.S. The NCPA describes itself on the Website as a "nonprofit, nonpartisan public policy research organization with the goal to develop and promote private alternatives to government regulation and control, solving problems by relying on the strength of the competitive, entrepreneurial private sector." Not surprisingly, then, the above document touts the private market place as the solution to health care problems of cost, access, and quality while avoiding evidence to the contrary. Many of the NCPA's "myths" have been rebutted in detail elsewhere as disinformation.[2]

Clearly the risk of basing national health policy on anything less than actual experience and well-grounded evidence is too high to accept. In an effort to disentangle rhetoric from reality and further rational discourse on health care reform, this chapter briefly considers some common myths about health care and health insurance.

Common Myths

1. Patients' appetites for health care are the main problem driving runaway health care costs; increased cost-sharing can therefore contain costs.

This is a pervasive view among health economists, most of whom have based the conventional theory of health insurance on "moral hazard." This theory dates back to a classic article by economist Mark Pauly in 1968.[3] By this they believe that health insurance provides a perverse incentive encouraging people with insurance to overuse health care services, thereby resulting in a "moral hazard welfare loss." Or, in other words, because people don't pay for health care directly, but their insurance pays, they will use it without regard to cost.

Economists, together with many health policy analysts and legislators, have therefore seen increases in cost-sharing with patients and their families as an essential way to rein in unnecessary care. The more patients pay, the more careful they will be in using health care. Indeed, this has become the conceptual lynch pin of consumer-directed health care (CDHC), currently the most politically popular approach to cost-containment. This statement by Senate Majority Leader Bill Frist in 2004 represents this approach, now being put forward as individual mandate legislation in many states.[4]

> *"The new [health care] system also must be responsive primarily to individual consumers, rather than to third-party payers. Most health care today is paid for and controlled by third parties, such as the government, insurers, and employers. A consumer-driven system will empower all people—if they so choose—to make decisions that will directly affect the most fundamental and intimate aspect of their life—their own health. This empowerment gives people a greater stake in, and more responsibility for, their own health care. Health care will not improve in a sustained and substantial way until consumers drive it."*

As proof of the moral hazard theory, economists point to a study conducted between 1974 and 1982 and published by RAND in 1993, the Rand Health Insurance Experiment (HIE). This is the only randomized experimental study of the relationship between health insurance and health to compare the effects of greater cost-sharing and no cost-sharing among insurance plans over many years. It found that HIE participants in high-deductible plans used 25 to 30 percent fewer service than those in the "free care," non-cost-sharing plan.[5]

Counter balanced against this single study that is over a decade old is growing evidence that other factors driving health care costs are far more important. These include technological advances, changing thresholds for defining "disease" (egs., osteoporosis and hyperlipidemia), increasing prevalence of chronic disease in an aging population, wasteful administrative costs in an inefficient system, high levels of *physician*-induced demand, and corporate profiteering throughout the medical-industrial complex. Of these, technology advances with a "medical arms race" among providers are especially costly. In addition, cost-sharing paradoxically leads not to consumers frugally reining in costs but to higher costs. Because they want to save money, patients skimp on necessary care, such as cutting back on expensive but important medications. In turn this can lead to worse health outcomes requiring greater interventions later at higher costs.[6,7]

The growing evidence that cost-sharing doesn't mean cost containment and in fact leads to many instances to adverse clinical outcomes has led Dr. John Nyman, health economist at the University of Minnesota, to reject the conventional theory of health insurance as "inefficient and welfare decreasing." He has assembled the evidence that shows that insured people are better off.[8,9]

Here are several examples among many studies that document the adverse outcomes of cost-sharing and discredit cost-sharing as a cost containment tool:

- A 2004 HIE study found that patients with hypertension who are both poor and sick have an annual likelihood of death 10 percent higher than for healthier and more affluent participants[10]
- Another RAND 2004 study found that doubling of co-payments led to less use of prescription drugs for diabetes (by 23 percent) and other chronic illnesses as well as a 17 percent increase in emergency room visits and a 10 percent increase in length of hospitalization[11]

- The 2003 Commonwealth Fund Biennial Health Insurance Survey found that patients with high deductibles forego necessary health care, as shown in Figure 4.1. Commonwealth Fund President Karen Davis points out that "the evidence is that increased patient cost-sharing leads to underuse of appropriate care."[12]

Figure 4.1

"Consumer-Driven" Plans = Worse Care
Patients with High Deductibles Forego Needed Care

Percent Failing to Get Needed...

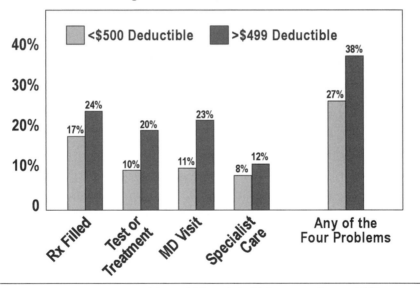

Source: Commonwealth Fund Biennal Health Insurance Survey, 2003

- A 2007 systematic review by investigators at RAND and the National Bureau of Economic Research assessed 132 articles published between 1985 and 2006 which examined associations between cost-sharing and use of prescription drugs; it found that increased cost-sharing is associated with such adverse events as increased use of ER visits and hospitalizations, together with worse clinical outcomes for patients with congestive heart failure, lipid disorders, diabetes, schizophrenia, and possibly asthma.[13]

- An Issue Paper by the Kaiser Commission on Medicaid and the Uninsured concluded that whatever cost "savings" are gained by cost-sharing are achieved at the expense of limiting necessary care.[14]

2. If people are uninsured, it's because they choose or prefer to go without insurance.

This is another myth popular among conservatives which holds that the uninsured lack enough responsibility to choose to insure themselves. But this view is untenable since the costs of health insurance have spiraled upward at a rate five times the inflation rate since 2000, so that health insurance has become unaffordable for a large part of the population. A report from the Commonwealth Fund in 2006 shows that uninsurance is now an All-American problem, with three in five Americans with annual incomes of $40,000 or more experiencing difficulties in paying medical bills or accrued debt. Figure 4.2 shows the percentage of uninsured by income level in 2004-2005.[15]

Figure 4.2

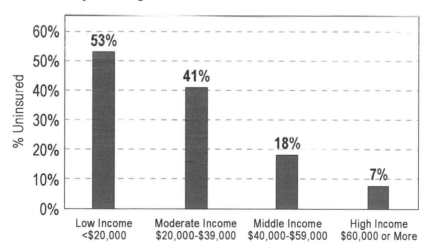

Without Health Insurance by Income Level, 2005*

Percent by Working Adults

*Currently uninsured, or uninsured at some time in the past year

Source: Collins S.R., Davis K., Doty M., Kriss J.L. & Holmgren A.L. "Gaps in Health Insurance: An All-American Problem." The Commonwealth Fund, Washington, DC, April 2006. Reprinted by permission.

More than four in five Americans without health insurance are employed but still can't afford health insurance. In fact, a 2006 report by Families USA found that a majority of more than 9 million uninsured children come from two-parent families with both parents working.[16] According to Woolhandler and Himmelstein's analysis of 2006 CPS data and federal poverty guidelines (set at about $20,000 for a family of 4), three quarters of the uninsured have incomes below 300 percent of those guidelines.[17] And as we saw in the last chapter, many low and middle-income workers can only afford limited benefit policies (LBPs) which offer little protection against the costs of any significant illness or injury.

3. The uninsured get care anyhow.

We do have a loosely woven patchwork of mostly public programs, including community health centers, urgent care clinics, emergency rooms, and local health departments reimbursed mostly by Medicaid and SCHIP. However, whatever safety net of public programs we once had is increasingly underfunded, fragile and unreliable. These examples show how tenuous this situation has become for many millions of Americans.

- A 2005 report from the Center for Studying Health System Change (HSC) found that the uninsured are as likely as the insured to perceive the need for care, but only half as likely to get care.[18]
- Another 2005 report of a national study of uninsured patients found that only one-quarter of them, after being seen in Emergency Rooms, were offered follow-up clinic appointments for urgent problems, even after they offered to pay $20 and arrange payments for the balance.[19]
- Although community health centers (CHCs) are an important resource of accessible and culturally sensitive care for underserved populations, they remain grossly underfunded and fall far short of the need; in 2004, for example, only $36 was allocated for each uninsured person receiving care in a CHC, and CHCs at that time provided care for only 20 percent of the nation's underserved and 10 percent of the uninsured.[20,21]

- Children with public or no insurance in Colorado, as well as nationally, have been found in a 2006 report to have higher severity of illness, higher mortality rates, and higher hospital charges.[22]
- A 2007 study by Public Citizen's Health Research Group reported that about 60 percent of poor Americans are not covered by Medicaid; eligibility and coverage policies vary widely from one state to another as many states obtain federal waivers;[23] Utah has eliminated Medicaid coverage of hospital and specialty care;[24] in order to qualify for Medicaid in Missouri, a family of three must have an annual income of no more than $3,504, less than one-quarter of the federal poverty level.[25]
- Coverage and eligibility policies for Medicaid will soon become even more stringent under new rules proposed by The Center for Medicare and Medicaid Services (CMS) in February 2008. These rules give states more control over their Medicaid benefit packages and greater latitude to impose increased cost-sharing on enrollees.[26]

4. Private health insurance provides more choice, efficiency, and value than one-size fits all government insurance.

Although the private health insurance industry continues to perpetuate this myth, its track record does not support this claim. We saw in the last chapter many examples of less choice and value of private plans even as their premiums become less affordable for much of the population. Figure 4.3 compares ratings of health insurance coverage by health status, income level and insurance coverage as determined by the 2001 Commonwealth Fund Health Insurance Survey—whether healthy or sick, higher or lower income, the results consistently favor traditional Medicare.[27] Another more recent study by the Commonwealth Fund showed than only 53 percent of employer-insured adults under age 65 are offered two or more choices of health plans, and that lower-income workers have the least choice.[28]

Likewise, comparisons of efficiency between private insurance plans and publicly-financed programs also leave little room for debate. Private insurers maximize profits by avoiding coverage of higher-risk

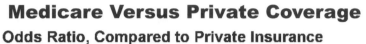

Figure 4.3

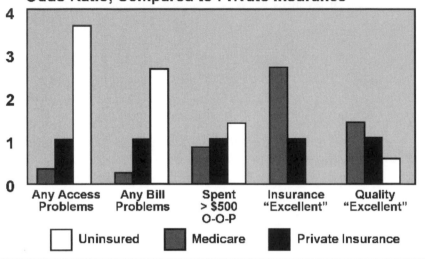

Medicare Versus Private Coverage
Odds Ratio, Compared to Private Insurance

| | Uninsured | Medicare | Private Insurance |

Source: Reprinted with permission from Davis K., Schoen C., Doty M., & Tenney K. Medicare versus private insurance: Rhetoric and reality. Health Affairs Web Exclusive W321, October 9, 2002.

groups and individuals through sharp underwriting and marketing. They are efficient—at generating returns for investors. But they are inefficient by carrying much higher overhead and staffing costs than public programs. That the motivation of private insurers is for profits more than service is illustrated by this statement by Dr. John Rowe in 2003 as chairman and CEO of Aetna, the nation's third largest private insurer:[29] "In 2002, Aetna improved its financial performance. This success was built on a seven-point reduction in the medical cost ratio (MCR), as well as lower administrative costs. This decline in MCR was driven by three factors: reduction of membership with historically higher MCRs, premium increases... and changing contracts and benefits."

Medicare is managed with an administrative overhead of about 3 percent compared to overhead costs of 19.9 percent for commercial carriers and 26.5 percent for investor-owned Blues.[30] In California, a 2005 study found that 22 percent of private health insurance premiums go to sales, marketing, billing, and other administrative tasks that are unnecessary in a publicly-financed program.[31]

5. The U.S. has the best health care system in the world.

It is true that the U.S. spends far more on health care than any other country in the world, and also has the most access to medical technologies. For many, that leads to a false assumption that our quality of care and health care system are world-beaters. However, there are many reports which refute this assumption, including the lack of improved outcomes in areas with more neonatologists and NICUs,[32] worse outcomes for seniors in areas with increased use of technology and specialist services,[33] and many other examples which confirm the risks and harms of more technological services.[34]

Cross-national comparisons for many years have consistently documented comparatively poor performance of our health care system compared to other industrialized countries around the world. There is no ambiguity in these reports.

- A 2000 report from the World Health Organization, based on such indicators as disability-adjusted life expectancy and child survival to five years of age, found the average ranking of the U.S. to be 15th out of 25 countries[35]
- A 2006 report found that Americans in late middle age are less healthy than their counterparts in Britain for diabetes, hypertension, heart disease, stroke, lung disease, and cancer [36]
- A 2007 study by the Commonwealth Fund, based on a survey of 12,000 adults in Australia, Canada, Germany, the Netherlands, New Zealand, the U.K., and the U.S., found that American adults encounter higher rates of medical errors, avoid essential care more often because of cost, have much greater difficulty in paying for necessary care, and are most likely to believe (34 percent) that their health care system needs to be completely rebuilt.[37]
- Another 2007 study found that Canada, although spending only about half on health care per capita as the U.S., has at least as good quality of care as this country, often with better health outcomes[38]
- A 2007 report ranked the U.S. 42nd in the world for life expectancy (behind Japan and most of Europe) and 41st in infant mortality rate (again worse than most of Europe, Cuba and Taiwan)[39]

- A 2008 report of a study of preventable deaths in 19 OECD countries (deaths that "should not occur in the presence of timely and effective health care") found that the U.S. ranks last in reducing these preventable deaths[40] (Figure 4.4)

All of these findings have led Ezekiel Emanuel, MD, PhD, of the Department of Clinical Bioethics at the National Institutes of Health, to this observation:[41]

Figure 4.4

Percentage Decline In Mortality From Amenable Causes And Other Causes Of Death Among Males Ages 0-74 In Nineteen Countries From 1997-98 To 2002-03

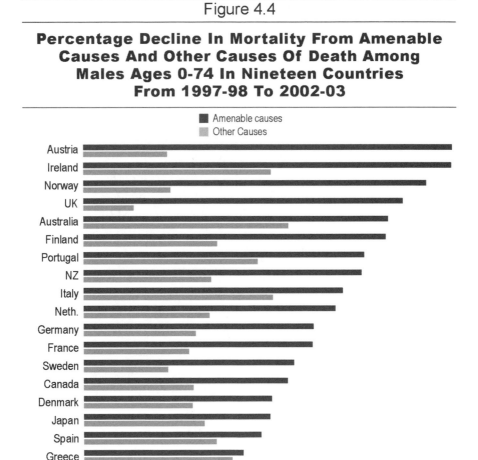

Source: Authors calculations based on data from the World Health Organization mortality database. Note: Denmark: 2000-02; Sweden: 2001-02, Italy, US: 2002
Reprinted with permission from Nolte E. & McKee C.M. Measuring the health of nations: Updating an earlier analysis. Health Aff 27(1):63,2008

"The U.S. health care system is considered a dysfunctional mess. Conventional wisdom has been turned on its head. If a politician declares that the United States has the best health care system in the world today, he or she looks clueless rather than patriotic or authoritative."

6. The U.S. health care system is mostly private

Many assume this to be the case since we have about 1,300 private health insurers entrenched in a private, market-based delivery system. Yet public financing supports a growing majority of health care spending. As we have already seen in Chapter 1, the federal Agency for Healthcare Research and Quality (AHRQ) estimates that the government finances 60 percent of the nation's annual health spending, including direct payments as well as subsidies for tax exemptions. These tax-free exemptions total $340 billion a year ($140 billion for employers offering employer-based health insurance and $200 billion for their covered employees).[42] To the 60 percent AHRQ estimate of public financing, Princeton health economist Uwe Reinhardt adds another 5 percent for the federal mandate that hospitals provide free care for the uninsured, so that the government actually pays for almost two-thirds of the nation's health care. In overview then, private health insurance covers (to an extent) about two-thirds of the U.S. population while paying for about one-third of total health expenditures.[43] In fact, by 1999 tax-financed health care expenditures in the U.S. exceeded total health care spending per capita in ten countries.[44]

7. The competitive marketplace will fix healthcare system problems of access, costs, and quality

Free markets have long been touted in this country as "the American way," to the point that markets are held up as both invincible and inevitable. A typical claim of market ideology in health care is illustrated by this statement by senior fellows at the Hoover Institution, a conservative think tank:[45]

"Greater reliance on individual choice and free markets are the solutions to what ails our health care system... A handful of policy changes that harness the power of markets for health services have the potential to give patients and their

*physicians more control over health-care choices, create more
health insurance options, lower health costs, reduce the number of uninsured persons—and give workers a pay increase to
boot."*

Despite this rhetoric, however, there is a long history of failures
of the private sector to improve system problems of access, cost, and
quality. There are many reasons why market theories don't apply in
health care. Here are some of the most important ones.

- A nine-year study by the Community Tracking Study of 12
  major U.S. health care markets found widespread skepti-
  cism that markets can improve efficiency and quality of the
  health care system; instead, it found these four barriers to
  efficiency: (1) providers' market power; (2) absence of potentially efficient provider systems; (3) employers' inability
  to push the system toward efficiency and quality; and (4)
  insufficient health plan competition.[46]
- Consolidation among providers limits choice and competition in many markets; in El Paso, Texas, for example, Tenet,
  the second largest hospital chain in the country, controls
  almost 80 percent of hospital beds.[47] One-half of Americans
  live in areas where the population is too small for any real
  competition; it is estimated that a metropolitan market of at
  least 400,000 is needed before there can be any chance of
  competition among facilities or providers.[48]
- A 2006 study by the AMA found near-monopolies by private
  insurers in 95 percent of HMO/PPO metropolitan markets,
  and that many markets exceeded thresholds that triggered
  antitrust concerns by the U.S. Department of Justice;[49] Figure 4.5 shows the extent of oligopoly among private health
  insurers.[50]
- In our deregulated marketplace, providers and facilities are
  often free to set their own prices; in California, for example,
  Tenet hospitals have been found by a state agency to charge
  60 to 90 percent higher than statewide averages for 7 common diagnoses,[51] as well as charges for drugs that were ten
  times the state averages.[52]

Figure 4.5

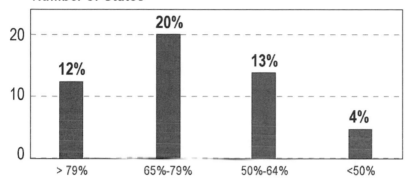

Health Insurance Oligopoly
A Few Plans Dominate Most States

Number of States

Market Share of 3 Largest Commercial Insurers

Source: Robinson, J.C. Consolidation and the transformation of competition in health insurance. *Health Affairs*, November/December 2004; 23(6): 11-24

- Our system is largely driven by acute illness, so that most visits for acute or semi-urgent problems are limited to providers and facilities within the community.
- Many people find it difficult to "shop" for medical care in our system with limited information on cost and quality; in addition, there are many subsets of the population, including the frail elderly, chronically ill and disabled, and those with language or literacy barriers, who are especially constrained in seeking out options among providers and facilities.

In recent years, the U.S. has been running what amounts to a giant experiment that reveals whether privatized health insurance is indeed more efficient and saves money. This has been the privatization of Medicare, from the HMOs of the 1990s to the HMO-PPOs and Part D Prescription Drug Benefit today. The results are devastating for the market enthusiasts on every front: our current privatized system as measured by efficiency, cost containment, improved access, value, or quality loses out when held up against publicly-financed Medicare as a governmental program.

The original hope for private Medicare programs was that they would offer more value and efficiency than traditional Medicare. For that reason, reimbursement was initially set at 95 percent of Medicare FFS reimbursement. Lobbying by industry was successful in resetting that figure in 1999 to well over 100 percent through a complex reimbursement formula which allowed rates up to 130 percent in some counties. Generous overpayments were continued through the 2003 Medicare legislation (MMA) so that today's averages are 112 to 119 percent of Medicare FFS (ie., 12 to 19 percent *less* efficient).

For all of these overpayments, which now amount to some $65 billion over the next 10 years, what do we get? These examples show how poorly privatized Medicare competes with traditional Medicare, even when the playing field is tilted in the private sector's favor.

- The MMA of 2003 expressly forbids CMS from using its bulk purchasing power to negotiate the prices of prescription drugs with manufacturers; the VA has done so for many years, achieving average discounts of about 45 percent.
- Of the $14 billion in spending for the Part D prescription drug benefit in 2006, 13 percent was taken up by administrative costs and profits by insurance companies offering the benefit; Medicare patients saved less than $9 a month compared to what they were spending for drugs before the benefit became available.[53]
- Between 1998 and 2000, when private Medicare + Choice HMOs were receiving an average of 113 percent reimbursement compared to FFS Medicare, many withdrew from the market when profits fell short of expectations, forcing 2.4 million seniors to find other coverage, and often requiring a change of physicians.[54]
- A 1999 national study found that investor-owned HMOs scored worse than not-for-profit plans on all 14 quality indicators reported to the National Committee for Quality Assurance (NCQA).[55]
- Humana, the second largest purveyor of private Medicare Advantage plans, was reprimanded by the Oklahoma State Insurance Commissioner in 2007 for widespread misconduct by its agents; misrepresentation of private Medicare

plans is a national problem as insurers promote their products with little federal oversight.[56]

• Both the General Accounting Office and the Office of Inspector General have already concluded that private Medicare plans are more expensive and less efficient than FFS Medicare, and in the long run threaten the fiscal sustainability of Medicare.[57,58] The Congressional Budget Office (CBO) reports that payments to private Medicare Advantage plans increased from $36 billion in 2004 to about $60 billion in 2006, and are projected to soar to $196 billion by 2017, far more than the projected costs of Original Medicare.[59]

• CMS is charged with monitoring the performance of Medical Advantage plans. A 2007 GAO report found that CMS examined just 14 percent of the plans in 2006, less than one-half the required number for oversight. These plans were contracted to spend money to provide additional benefits, and lower co-payments or premiums in 2003. The GAO study found that they fell short of what they were contracted to spend by $35 million.[60]

• A 2008 GAO report found that more than one-half of the 8 million enrollees in Medicare Advantage plans are in plans without an annual limit on out-of-pocket spending for medical care (ie., no protection against high medical bills).[61]

• Perhaps most importantly and tragically, the inefficiency is not the worst of it. Health outcomes for enrollees in private Medicare plans are at their lowest level since quality reporting was begun in 1998, and they compare poorly with other health plans; from 2005 to 2006, data collected by the National Committee for Quality Assurance (NCQA) showed that private Medicare plans improved on only 7 of 38 reporting measures compared to 30 of 44 measures for commercial plans and 34 of 43 measures for private Medicaid plans.[62] Privatization has clearly come to mean paying more to get less.

The above experience of the private marketplace at work shows that this observation by Joseph Stiglitz, Nobel laureate in economics and former chief economist of the World Bank, is right on target: [63]

> *"Markets do not lead to efficient outcomes, let alone outcomes that comport with social justice. As a result, there is often good reason for government intervention to improve the efficiency of the market. Just as the Great Depression should have made it evident that the market often does not work as well as its advocates claim, our recent Roaring Nineties should have made it self-evident that the pursuit of self-interest does not necessarily lead to overall economic efficiency."*

8. Government-financed health care could not provide adequate coverage and quality of care at an affordable cost

We are now living in a time when many Americans have little faith in the capacity of government to do important work well. Indeed, the government's response to Hurricane Katrina, marred as it was by incompetence, poor coordination, and cronyism, lends credibility to that belief. This country has also had an ongoing debate over the role of government since its founding. Commentator and author Jim Hightower brings this historical perspective to the debate:[64]

> *"Granted, people (including me) don't like Big Government, but as we learned from Bush's Katrina fiasco, we damned sure do want essential government. This has been the case from the start of our nation, and the boneheaded, shortsighted, self-aggrandizing, "kill government" ideologues of today are enemies of history, common sense, progress, and America's public welfare.*
>
> *The first W—George Washington—was on board with using public funds to provide the new country with a solid infrastructure, including an extensive system of postal roads and canals. Jefferson stepped up with tax dollars for the Louisiana Purchase. Even in a time of civil war, Honest Abe saw the need for a transcontinental railroad, the Homestead Act, and a public system of land-grant colleges. Teddy Roosevelt—a Republican—pushed for our sterling network of national parks and created the National Forest Service. FDR put America to work building courthouses and dams, planting windbreaks and*

arbors, creating music and plays—jewels that are still with us. Ike, a fiscal conservative, saw the need to launch the Interstate Highway System. Lyndon Johnson fought for crucial investments in hospitals, schools, water systems, and parks."

As Hightower points out, the U.S. has a long history of massive yet successful government programs.

As one-sixth of the nation's GDP, the U.S. health care system is certainly a big challenge requiring a high degree of competence, commitment, and accountability to resolve its increasing problems. But we already have two well-established examples of such competence—traditional FFS Medicare and the Veterans Administration—which have shown superior performance compared to the private sector for many years. Their track records speak for themselves.

Medicare's strength as a publicly-financed program has been based for more than 40 years on its universality, shared risk, dependability, and relative administrative simplicity. Now covering 42 million senior and disabled Americans, the program guarantees access to a broad range of services to all enrollees, as well as free choice of physician and hospital. Its coverage is rated higher than private insurers (Figure 4.3), and it has been more effective in cost containment over the last 30 years than the private sector.[65] As argued elsewhere,[66] the program could provide even more value if corporate profiteering, administrative complexity, and waste of private plans were reduced or eliminated together with other value-based reforms, such as applying cost effectiveness in coverage decisions and filling some gaps in essential services. Despite its problems, however, Medicare has been shown to decrease, or even reverse, health disparities after previously uninsured people with chronic illness become eligible for the program at age 65, thereby gaining improved access to essential care.[67]

The VA system gives another example of a strong public program with a superior track record compared to private plans. With its 154 hospitals and 875 clinics across the country, the VA serves 5.4 million patients, double the number 10 years ago. The VA system has been more effective than private plans in improving quality of care, containing costs, and application of electronic records. Table 4.1 shows how the quality of care in VA hospitals compares with non-VA hospitals, based on studies by RAND and AHRQ.[68] Many other studies have demonstrated better quality of care by the VA in selected areas, such as control of diabetes[69] and care for patients with heart attacks.[70]

Table 4.1

Quality of Care in VA Versus Non-VA Hospitals

Health Indicator	VA Score*	National Sample**
Overall	67%	51%
Chronic care	72%	59%
Lung disease	69%	59%
Heart disease	73%	70%
Depression	80%	62%
Diabetes	70%	47%
Hypertension	78%	65%
High cholesterol	64%	53%
Osteoarthritis	65%	57%
Preventive care	64%	44%
Acute care	53%	55%
Screening	68%	46%
Diagnosis	73%	61%
Treatment	56%	41%
Follow-up	73%	58%

* 596 VA patients ** 992 patients at non-VA hospitals
Data: RandCorp; Agency for Healthcare Research & Quality

Source: Arnst, C. The best medical care in the U.S. *Business Week*, July 17, 2006

Why Do These Myths Matter?

The above myths, despite their lack of factual basis, are important because they allow market advocates to perpetuate the status quo and avoid rational public debate over health care policy. George Lakoff, Professor of Linguistics at the University of California Berkeley reminds us in his book *Don't Think Of an Elephant!: Know Your Values and Frame the Debate---The Essential Guide for Progressives* of the importance of framing issues based upon values and facts. Opponents of any form of publicly financed health insurance have for many years successfully used these myths to frame this debate based on their version of personal responsibility, individualism and American exceptionalism without any regard for egalitarian values or the failures of markets.

We have not yet had a rational evidence-based debate in this country over policy alternatives to address the growing and already unacceptable problems of our health care system. Instead, we have a short-sighted polarized "debate" with excess rhetoric and disinformation easily manipulated to obfuscate the real issues and avoid health care reform. Meanwhile, the real issues, such as the role of government, whether private health insurance serves the public interest, and whether health care is just another commodity to be bought and sold on an open market, are being sidestepped.

As our system further deteriorates and reform becomes more urgent, the real issues need to be reframed based upon experience, values, and evidence, not myths, smoke and mirrors. Dr. Don McCanne offers us this example of reframing in his recent rebuttal to the common argument by conservatives for HSAs and more responsible choices by patients in a system of consumer-directed health care:[71]

> *"The wealthiest nation of all is not financially equipped to do what all other industrialized nations have – insuring everyone? And the fear of spending money from a health savings account is a greater incentive to quit smoking than the fear of cancer, heart disease or emphysema? Get real! We each have a personal responsibility to take care of ourselves, but we also have an egalitarian responsibility to our fellow Americans to see that financial hardship does not compound the misfortune of illness or injury."*

These first four chapters have examined the history, claims, and actual track record of the private health insurance industry in the U.S. In the next chapter, we will consider whether it is equipped and qualified to remain as a major financing base for our failing health care system.

References

1. Goodman J.C. & Herrick D.M. *Twenty Myths about Single-Payer Health Insurance: International Evidence on the Effects of National Health Insurance in Countries Around the World.* National Center for Policy Analysis, Dallas, 2002.
2. Geyman J.P. Myths and memes about single-payer health insurance in the United States: A rebuttal to conservative claims. *Int J Health Serv* 35 (1): 53-60, 2005.
3. Pauly M.V. The economics of moral hazard: Comment. *Am Econ Rev* 58(3):1968.
4. Frist W.H. Health care in the 21st century. N Engl J Med 352:267-72, 2004.
5. Newhouse J. P., and the Insurance Experiment Group. *Free for All: Lessons from the RAND Health Insurance Experiment.* Cambridge, MA, Harvard University Press, 1993.
6. Newhouse J.P. Consumer-directed health plans and the RAND health insurance experiment. *Health Aff (Millwood)* 23(6):107-13, 2004.
7. Soumerai S.B., Ross-Degnan D., Avorn J., McLaughlin T. J. & Choodnovskkiy I. Effects of Medicaid drug-payment limits on admission to hospitals and nursing homes. *N Engl J Med* 325:1072-77, 2004.
8. Nyman J.A. *The Theory of Demand for Health Insurance.* Stanford, CA, Stanford University Press, 2003.
9. Nyman J.A. Is "moral hazard" inefficient? The policy implications of a new theory. *Health Aff (Millwood)* 23(5):194-99, 2004.
10. Ibid #6.
11. Goldman D.P., et al. Pharmacy benefits and the use of drugs by the chronically ill. *JAMA* 291:2344-2350, 2004.
12. Davis K. *Half of Insured Adults with High-Deductible Health Plans Experience Medical Bill or Debt Problems.* New York, Commonwealth Fund, January 27, 2005.
13. Goldman D.P., Joyce G.F.,& Zheng Y. Prescription drug cost sharing: Associations with medication and medical utilization and spending and health. *JAMA* 298 (11):61-88, 2007.
14. Artiga S. & O"Malley M. Increasing premiums and cost sharing in Medicaid and SCHIP: Recent state experiences. Issue Paper. Kaiser Commission on Medicaid and the Uninsured. Kaiser Family Foundation, May 2005, p 2.
15. Collins S.R., Davis K., Doty M., Kriss J.L. & Holmgren A.L. Gaps in Health Insurance: An All-American Problem. The Commonwealth Fund, Washington, DC, April 2006.
16. Families USA. Press release. New report: Majority of uninsured children live in two-parent families. Washington, D,C., September 25, 2006.
17. Woolhandler S. & Himmelstein D. U. Income distribution of the uninsured. Chicago, IL: Physicians for a National Health Program, 2006.
18. Hadley J., & Cunningham P. J. Perception, reality and health insurance: Uninsured as likely as insured to perceive need for care but half as likely to get care. Washington, D.C.: Center for Studying Health System Change, Issue Brief

#100, October 2005.

19. Asplin B.R., Rhodes K.V., Levy H., et al. Insurance status and access to urgent ambulatory care follow-up appointments. *JAMA* 294(10):1248-54, 2005.

20. National Association of Community Health Centers. With new census figures, community health centers brace for more uninsured patients: Health centers already struggling with more patients, less resources. Available from: URL: http://www.nachc.com/press/newcensus.asp.2003.

21. Schiff G. & Fegan C. Community health centers and the underserved: Eliminating disparities or increasing despair. *J Health Policy* 24(3/4):44-7, 2004.

22. Todd J., Armon C., Griggs A., Poole S. & Berman S. Increased rates of morbidity, mortality and charges for hospitalized children with public or no health insurance in Colorado and the United States. *Pediatrics* August 2006.

23. Public Citizen. Unsettling scores: A ranking of State Medicaid programs. *Health Letter* 23(4):April 2007.

24. Pear R. *New York Times*, January 19, 2005.

25. Solomon D. Wrestling with Medicaid cuts. *Wall Street Journal*, February 16, 2006:A4.

26. Centers for Medicare and Medicaid Services (CMS). CMS Proposes New Rules for Redesigning Medicaid States Have Greater Flexibility in Benefits, Cost Sharing, February 21, 2008.

27. Davis K., Schoen C., Doty M., & Tenney K. Medicare versus private insurance: Rhetoric and reality. *Health Affairs Web Exclusive* W321, October 9, 2002.

28. Commonwealth Fund. Many with insurance lack choice. New York: Issue Brief, 2005.

29. Aetna. Aetna reports fourth quarter and full-year 202 results. Press release. Feb. 11, 2003.

30. Himmelstein D. U. The National Health Program Slide-Show Guide. Center for National Health Program Studies. Cambridge, Mass: 2000.

31. Kahn J.G., Kronick R., Kryer M., & Gans D. N. The cost of health insurance administration in California: Estimates for insurers, physicians, and hospitals. *Health Aff (Millwood)* 24:6, 2005.

32. Thompson L.A., Goodman D.C., & Little G.A. Is more neonatal intensive care always better? Insights from a cross-national comparison of reproductive care. *Pediatrics* 109:1036-43, 2002.

33. Wennberg J.B., Fisher E.S. & Skinner J.S. Geography and the debate over Medicare reform. *Health Affairs Web Exclusive* W-103, February 13, 2002.

34. Fisher E.S. & Welch H.G. Avoiding the unintended consequences of growth in medical care: How might more be worse? *JAMA* 281:446-53, 1999.

35. World Health Report 2000. Available at http://www.who.int/whr/000en/report.htm.

36. Banks J., Marmot M., Oldfield Z., & Smith J.P. Disease and disadvantage in the United States and in England. *JAMA* 295:2037-45, 2006.

37. Schoen C., Osborn R., Doty M., Bishop M, Peugh J. & Murukutia N. Toward higher-performance health system adults' health care experiences in seven countries, 2007. *Health Aff Web Exclusive* October 31, 2007.

38. Guyatt G.H., Devereaux P.J., Lexchin J., Stone S.B., Yalnizyan A., Himmelstein D,U. & Woolhandler S., et al. A systematic review of studies comparing health outcomes in Canada and the United States. *Open Medicine* 1(1): 2007.
39. Associated Press. U.S. ranks just 42nd in life expectancy. Lack of insurance, obesity, social disparities to blame experts say. August 11, 2007.
40. Nolte E. & McKee C.M. Measuring the health of nations: Updating an earlier analysis. *Health Aff* 27(1):63, 2008.
41. Emanuel E. J. What cannot be said on television about health care. *JAMA* 297(19):2131-3, 2007.
42. Editorial. Health care by loopholes. *AARP Bulletin* 48(3):3, 2007.
43. Gross D. National health care? We're halfway there. *New York Times*, December 3, 2006.
44. Woolhandler S., & Himmelstein D. U. Paying for national health insurance—and not getting it. *Health Aff (Millwood)* 21(4):93, 2002.
45. Cogan J.F., Hubbard R.G. & Kessler D.P. Keep government out. *Wall Street Journal,* January 13, 2006;A12.
46. Nichols L.M., et al. Are market forces strong enough to deliver efficient health care systems? Confidence is waning. *Health Aff (Millwood)* 23(2):8-21, 2004.
47. Stein L. Pulling the plug. *Metro.* Silicon's Valley weekly newspaper, September 20, 2002.
48. Kronick R., Goodman D.C., Weinberg J., & Wagner E. The marketplace in health care reform. The demographic limitations of managed competition. *N Engl J Med* 328:148, 1993.
49. Associated Press. Study: Health insurers are near monopolies. April 18, 2006.
50. Robinson J.C. Consolidation and the transformation of competition in health insurance. *Health Aff* 23(6):11-24 2004.
51. Rapaport L. Tenet's fees for Medicare tops in state. *Sacramento Bee.* Retrieved from sacbee.com. November 27, 2002.
52. Abelson R. Nurses' Association says in study that big hospital chain overcharges patients for drugs. *The New York Times*, November 24, 2002.
53. Medicare Rights Center. What a waste. Asclepios 8(2) January 10, 2008.
54. Achman L. & Gold M. *New Analysis Describes 2004 Payment Increases to Medicare Advantage Plans.* Mathematica Policy Research, Washington, D.C., April 2004.
55. Himmelstein D.U., Woolhandler S., Hellander I., & Wolfe S. M. Quality of care in investor-owned vs. not-for-profit HMOs. *JAMA* 282(2):159-63, 1999.
56. Pear R. Insurer faces reprimand in Medicare marketing case. *New York Times*, May 15, 2007:A14.
57. General Accounting Office. *Medicare + Choice: Payments Exceed Costs of Fee for Service Benefits, Adding Billions to Spending.* GAO/HEHS-00-161 Washington, D.C.: Government Printing Office, 2000.
58. Jost T.S. Disentitlement? The Threats Facing Our Public Health Care Programs and a Rights-Based Response. New York: Oxford University Press, 2003, 113, citing multiple reports from the Office of Inspector General (OIG) 1997 to 2000 and related documents.

59. Orszag P.R. Testimony on the Medicare Advantage Program before the Committee on the Budget U.S. House of Representatives, June 28, 2007.
60. GAO. Medicare Advantage: Required Audits of Limited Value. U.S. Government Accountability Office, July 30, 2007.
61. GAO. Medicare Advantage: Increased spending relative to Medicare fee-for-service may not always reduce beneficiary out-of-pocket costs. Government Accountability Office, February 2008.
62. Medicare Rights Center. MEDPAC: private plan enrollees in poorer health. New York: *Medicare Watch* 10(24): November 27, 2007.
63. Stiglitz J.E. Evaluating economic change, *Daedalus* 133/3. Summer 2004.
64. Hightower J., & Frazer P. All in the name of killing government. Terrorists? Nope, it's Bush & Co. who"ve blasted our infrastructure. *The Hightower Lowdown* 8(11):2, 2006.
65. Boccuti C. & Moon M. Comparing Medicare and private insurers: Growth rates in spending over three decades. *Health Aff (Millwood)* 22(2):235, 2003.
66. Geyman J.P. *Shredding the Social Contract: The Privatization of Medicare.* Monroe, ME: Common Courage Press, 213-19, 2006.
67. McWilliams J.M., Meara E., Zaslavsky A.M. & Ayanian J.Z. Health of previously uninsured adults after acquiring Medicare coverage. *JAMA* 298(24):2881-94, 2007.
68. Arnst C. The best medical care in the US. *Business Week*, July 17, 2006.
69. Kerr E.A., Gerzoff R.B., Krein S.L., Selby J.V., Piette. J.D., et al. Diabetes care quality in the Veterans Affairs Health Care System and commercial managed care: The TRIAD study. *Ann Intern Med* 141(4):272-81, 2004.
70. Peterson L.A., Normand S.L., Leape L. L., & McNeil B. J. Comparison of use of medications after acute myocardial infarction in the Veterans Health Administration and Medicare. *Circulation* 104(24):2898-904, 2001.
71. McCanne D. Available at quote-of-the-day@mccanne.org, December 20, 2006 and http://www.memac.com/menag/article/articleDetail.jsp?id=390156.

CHAPTER 5

Terminally Ill: An Imploding Industry on a Death March

"Having committed ourselves irrevocably to voluntary health insurance, it is clearly up to the medical profession to provide a truly satisfactory medical security program. It would be fatal to fall too far short of this goal. If we succeed merely in giving everyone a partial and inadequate coverage, we will only aggravate the demand for a comprehensive governmental system."
—Dr. James Bryan
New Jersey Blue Shield Plan administrator, 1954[1]

"The state's private-sector health care market is in deep trouble and could implode unless all the players collaborate to provide coverage for the uninsured and reduce costs that are sending premiums skyward. Without action to overcome the problems of cost and access, the market will get to the point where the balance of power will move from the private market to the halls of government. And when that happens, it's hard to know what the solution coming out the door will look like."
—Bruce Bodaken, CEO of Blue Shield of California, 2005[2]

"American health insurance is experiencing a steady erosion—a death march as Americans find it increasingly difficult to afford the ever-rising tab for health insurance and medical services. The epicenter of this transformation is the crumbling of America's employment-based system of health financing, which arose in the mid-twentieth century as a distinctive response to the challenge of health insecurity in the United States. As health care costs have exploded in an increasingly competitive business environment, this old, odd bargain has

come undone—and the Great Risk Shift has relentlessly played out."

—Jacob Hacker, PhD[3]

Professor of Political Science, Yale University and Author of *The Great Risk Shift: The Assault on American Jobs, Families, Health Care and Retirement, and How You Can Fight Back*

The above three quotes, spanning more than half a century, show that we are on a moving train headed in the direction of disaster. Dr. Bryan's hope that the source to "provide a truly satisfactory medical security program" would spring from the medical profession has long since vanished, as was documented in my recent book *The Corrosion of Medicine: Can The Profession Reclaim Its Moral Legacy?*[4] As we have seen, the private sector has also failed to make health care more affordable. And in the last few years, the industry's death march has begun.

This chapter has two goals: (1) to examine the factors that have led to the industry's death march; and (2) to briefly summarize the reasons why we should discard private multi-payer financing of our health care system.

Major Factors in the Industry's Downhill Course

In previous chapters, we have touched on many egregious aspects of the health insurance industry that are costly or even detrimental to the health of patients. How do these play out as factors driving the death march? These eight factors answer this question.

Factor 1: Uncontrolled Inflation of Health Care Costs

As we have already seen, neither the medical profession nor any initiatives to date by the private sector or government have had any lasting success in containing runaway costs of health care in this country. We are now spending more than $2.3 trillion a year on health care (16.6 percent of GDP), about $7,800 per capita, and far more than other industrialized countries. Private health insurance costs are increasing by 6.7 percent a year while out-of-pocket payments grow by 6.1 percent, more than double the rise in the cost-of-living. These rates are expected to increase at about the same rate for the next decade, reaching 19.6 percent of GDP by 2016.[5,6]

There are many drivers to health care inflation, especially in a relatively unfettered market system. As previously discussed, these include the ability of manufacturers and suppliers in many instances to set their own prices, and the large amount of unnecessary services being provided by health professionals. But a major factor driving inflation is the inefficiency and waste of a private insurance industry taking up 31 percent of health care spending.

Despite the claims of market advocates that competition in an open marketplace will contain costs, this hope has been proven incorrect in health care.[7-9] The market has failed to contain health care spending, and current efforts to shift increased costs to patients and their families only lessen their ability to afford necessary care.[10-12] For this reason, other industrialized nations have all found it necessary to adopt one or another form of publicly-financed health insurance in order to rein in costs and to meet the needs of their populations. Public programs of universal coverage in other industrialized countries have contained costs much more effectively than in this country without restricting access to necessary services.[13]

Factor 2: Growing Unaffordability of Premiums and Health Care

Beyond lower-income people, the broad middle class is now having increasing difficulty affording either insurance or medical bills. The costs of health insurance premiums alone have far outstripped overall inflation and the growth in workers' earnings for most of the last 20 years, making health care progressively more unaffordable for a growing population of Americans.[14] The average family premium for employer-based coverage was $11,500 in 2006, an increase of 87 percent between 2000 and 2006 (Figure 5.1).[15] Almost one-half of Americans earn less than $30,000 a year[16] Even among adults with annual incomes between $50,000 and $75,000, one-third have serious problems paying for care.[17]

The costs of health insurance premiums, of course, have little to do with the total costs of health care as cost-sharing and out-of-pocket spending continue to increase for enrollees and as the benefits of insurance coverage decrease. A 2007 national survey of insured Americans

Figure 5.1

Cumulative Changes in Health Insurance Premiums, Overall Inflation, and Workers Earnings, 2000-2006

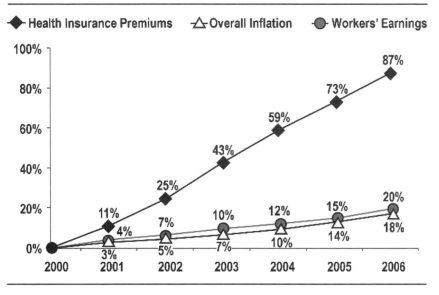

Note: Data on premium increases reflect the cost of health insurance premiums for a family of four. Source: KFF/HRET Survey of Employer-Sponsored Health Benefits, 2001-2006; Bureau of Labor Statistics, Consumer Price Index, U.S. City Average of Annual Inflation (April to April), 2001-2006; Bureau of Labor Statistics, Seasonally Adjusted Data from the Current Employment Statistics Survey (April to April), 2001-2006. This information was reprinted with permission from the Henry J. Kaiser Family Foundation. The Kaiser Family Foundation, based in Menlo Park, California, is a non-profit, private operating foundation focusing on the major health care issues facing the nation and is not associated with Kaiser Permanente or Kaiser Industries.

by *Consumer Reports* found that 29 percent of respondents were so underinsured that they postponed medical care because of costs and 43 percent were "somewhat" or "completely" unprepared to cope with a costly medical emergency over the coming year.[18] A 2007 study by the Commonwealth Fund found that adult women less than age 65, because of their greater health care needs and rates of use, are especially impacted by medical bills. Even with private insurance, it found that 50 percent of women between 19 and 64 years of age spend more than 10 percent of their income on out-of-pocket expenses and are more likely than men to avoid needed care.[19] A 2007 study by Georgetown University and the Kaiser Family Foundation found that pregnant women face high out-of-pocket costs under high-deductible health plans and that HSAs are not likely to help much. These costs now run from $5,000 to almost $8,000 for small group and individual market CDHPs and up to $20,000 and more for pregnancy complicated by gestational diabetes, pre-term labor, and C-section delivery.[20]

With near stagnant income and steadily rising household debt, middle-income families, struggling to buy and keep a home and save for retirement, are accumulating debt at an ever more rapid rate (Figure 5.2).[21] Average household credit card debt has more than doubled since 1994 as the average American now carries seven credit and debit cards.[22] A recent study of economic mobility conducted by several U.S. think tanks, including the Pew Charitable Trusts and the Brookings Institution, found that the median income for a man in his 30s in 2004 was $35,010, 12 percent *less* than that for men in his father's generation in 1974, adjusted for inflation.[23]

Difficult as the situation is for lower and middle-income Ameri-

Figure 5.2

Real Median Household Net Worth, Debt and Income, in 2000 Dollars

Consumers seized on low interest rates to buy new homes and refinance old home loans. Households debt outpaced wealth as income remained flat.

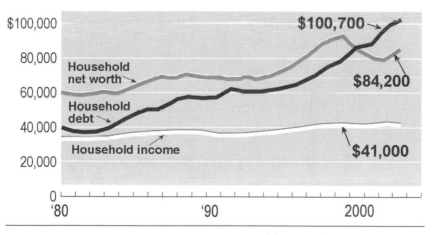

Sources: Federal Reserve Board, Economy.com, Freddie Mac, Bloomberg.
Reprinted with permission from: Henderson N. Greenspan's mixed legacy: America prospered during the Fed chiefs tenure, but built up massive debt. *Washington Post National Weekly Edition.* January 30-February 5, 2006, p 6.

cans, it will only get worse. Price Waterhouse Coopers' projections for health care costs in 2008 estimate that PPOs and HMOs will go up by 9.9 percent while CDHC plans will rise by 7.4 percent, again way beyond cost-of-living and earnings.[24] Hewitt Associates expects an even higher cost increase for HMOs in 2008 (14.1 percent).[25] Future years are even more worrisome. Princeton health economist Uwe Reinhardt notes that with an average premium increase of 8 to 10 percent over the next 10 years, premiums, deductibles, and co-payments will come to $21,000 a year for the average family by 2015.[26] And of course, as we saw in Chapter 1, annual health insurance premiums, as they continue to rise at rates well beyond earnings and inflation rates, will consume *all* of household income by 2025! (Figure 1.4).[27] Clearly the brick wall of reality will stop this cycle well before that time.

Factor 3: Decreasing Levels of Insurance Coverage

Having health insurance, whether private or public, means less all the time in terms of breadth, reliability, and value of coverage. Even as premiums go up, coverage goes down. Examples abound:

- A 2005 national study by the American Diabetes Association and Georgetown University found that people with diabetes encounter all kinds of problems with their coverage, including policies that exclude coverage, unaffordable premium increases, underwriting policies designating diabetes as "uninsurable," and high-risk pools excluding diabetes as a pre-existing condition.[28]
- A 2006 national study of people with cancer by the Kaiser Family Foundation and the Harvard School of Public Health found that even with consistent health insurance, one in five patients with cancer used up most or all of their life savings.[29]
- Stand-alone drug plans offering "doughnut hole" coverage of prescription drugs for Medicare patients will become more expensive, or disappear entirely, over the next few years; by 2013, the coverage gap of the doughnut hole will almost double from $2,850 in 2006 to $5,066 in 2013, within which seniors will have to bear all of their costs of prescription drugs. Premiums for these plans increased by a national average of 87 percent in 2007.[30]

- The limited benefit plans (LBPs) now being promoted by the insurance industry offer little more than the illusion of coverage, with annual caps as low as $1,000 to $2,500 and other restrictions. Many large insurers, including Aetna, Cigna, and BCBS, together with several smaller insurers, are seeing a lucrative new market, especially among an estimated 39 percent of employers who don't offer health insurance to their employees. In some cases, payments in premiums exceed the amounts received in actual benefits.[31]

An interesting recent study examined trends in affordability and comprehensiveness of small-group and individual insurance markets in California. "*Actuarial value*" was defined as "the proportion of claims expenses for covered services paid by the insurance plan for a large standardized population." From 2003 to 2006, the actuarial value in the small-group market was stable at 0.83 (83 percent of medical bills paid) while the actuarial value of individual plans fell dramatically from 0.75 to 0.55. The investigators concluded that out-of-pocket expenses in an unreformed individual market would be "catastrophic costs" to people of average means.[32]

As the debate over insurance coverage and health care costs continues, many place false emphasis upon insurance premiums without regard to out-of-pocket expenses for health care. Definition of underinsurance is essential to this debate. Researchers at the Commonwealth Fund offer us a useful definition of underinsurance as people who are insured all year but report at least one of these three indicators: "(1) Medical expenses amounted to 10 percent of income or more; (2) among low-income adults (below 200 percent of the federal poverty level), medical expenses amounted to at least 5 percent of income; and (3) health plan deductibles equaled or exceeded 5 percent of income."[33]

As the State of Massachusetts grapples with how to implement the 2006 individual mandate legislation, a 2007 study put numbers on how unaffordable the combination of insurance premiums and out-of-pocket expenses will be for many Massachusetts residents. Across all income groups, individuals and families with non-group coverage spent 16.9 percent and 14.7 percent of income, respectively, on premiums and out-of-pocket costs; for employer coverage, spending for these costs were 12.3 percent and 15.1 percent of income for individual and family coverage, respectively.[34]

By way of comparison in considering the financial burdens placed on individuals and families by medical costs, we need to remind ourselves that people 65 years of age and older spent 15 percent of their annual household income on premiums and out-of-pocket costs in 1965 when Medicare was enacted; that number had gone up to 22 percent by 2000,[35,36] and by 2003 one in four seniors on Medicare were spending at least 29.9 percent of their income on health care.[37]

American families with health insurance are increasingly vulnerable to heavy cost burdens as premiums and out-of-pocket expenses continue to rise at rates several times their incomes and cost-of-living. Having insurance provides less security each year against high cost burdens. A recent national study by the Lewin Group projected that 50 million non-elderly Americans will spend more than 10 percent of their pre-tax income on health care in 2008. More than three out of four people in families spending over 25 percent of their pre-tax income on health care are insured.[38]

This trend is disturbing. Once, just a few years ago, the alarm bells were rung over the number of people in this country who didn't have health insurance, people who faced a public safety net increasingly in tatters. I wrote a book on the subject to do my part of alarm-bell ringing, *Falling Through the Safety Net: Americans Without Health Insurance*.[39] Today, even those who are employed and insured with hard earned cash are falling through similar holes.

Factor 4: Fragmentation and Inefficiency

As we have seen in earlier chapters, the private health insurance industry fragments the risk pool among some 1,300 different insurers, all competing to sign up lower-risk enrollees in order to keep their medical-loss ratios as low as possible (ie., keep their payments for patient care services to a minimum while maximizing profits and returns for shareholders). Even as the industry encounters obstacles to further growth, its administrative bureaucracy continues to expand at a rapid rate. In a hallmark of inefficiency, for example, while its market fell by 1 percent between 2000 and 2005, its workforce grew by one-third.[40] Redundancy and inefficiency pervades this workforce, which is largely involved in marketing to healthier enrollees, underwriting and re-underwriting, and denial of coverage.

As noted earlier, this increasingly desperate cream-skimming defeats the primary function of insurance—to share risk through a broad risk pool—while increasing costs and shifting risk and costs to other people and institutions.

Two examples expose the inefficiencies of this bureaucracy. A study of 2,000 depressed patients in the Seattle area found that they were covered by 189 different plans with 755 different policies.[41] According to Dr. Allan Korn, medical director of the Chicago-based Blue Cross Blue Shield Association, Chicago has 17,000 different plan designs.[42] Is this maze what proponents of private insurance mean when they talk about "choice"?

In effect then, private insurers don't compete with each other by delivering better care at lower cost. That would be in line with what is understood as a classical form of competition where the consumer comes out on top. Insurance competition is different: who can avoid the most enrollees with higher medical costs, and who is most effective at delaying or denying payment when they can?[43]

Private insurers are not evil, they are just applying good business principles in an effort to avoid adverse risk selection, the great fear throughout the industry. In order to deal with increasing costs of sicker patients, insurers are forced to raise their premiums. If they attract too many higher-risk patients, these rate hikes can lead them into a "death spiral" where their rates are too high to maintain market share as healthier enrollees leave for lower cost plans.

The same pressures also apply to managed care organizations, even those that are not-for-profit. As a successful pioneer of a large integrated managed care organization for more than 60 years, Kaiser Permanente, which delivers comprehensive care for many of its subscribers over their entire lives, is now facing adverse selection within its aging population. Kaiser was the last large insurer to add deductibles to its plans in the individual (non-employer-based) market. It was forced to do so by market pressures, particularly from Blue Cross Blue Shield and other competitors who were flooding the market with low-premium-high deductible plans that undercut prices at the expense of quality.[44]

Factor 5: Shrinking Private Health Insurance Markets

The shift by employers away from financing the costs of health insurance has been dramatic. As we saw in Chapter 1, private employer sponsored insurance (ESI) arose as an "accidental system" of financing U.S. health care during the wartime years of the 1940s. It flourished for the next 30 years or so during times when American business was dominant, with few concerns about global competition, and when the labor movement was stronger than today. Since the 1980s, ESI has been in steady decline. From 1988 to 2004, the proportion of employers with 200 or more employees offering retiree health coverage dropped from two-thirds to just more than one-third.[45] Since 2000, the proportion of employers that finance the full cost of coverage, the norm in earlier years, dropped from 29 percent to 17 percent for individual coverage and from 11 percent to only 6 percent for family coverage.[46] By 2005, the proportion of Americans covered by ESI dropped to 59.5 percent, down from 63.6 percent in 2000.[47]

A 2006 report from the Kaiser Family Foundation cites several reasons for the continued decline of ESI in recent years:[48] "The first and most commonly discussed is that the rapid growth in health care premiums led to declines in employers offering health benefits, as well as the rate of which employees participate or 'take-up' these offers. But there are also demographic and workplace changes that affected the rate of employer-sponsored insurance. For example, in the past five years, there has been a shift towards work in small firms and to self-employment. There has also been a decline in employment in industries that have historically provided high rates of coverage and a substantial increase in employment in industries that have not."

Besieged as they are by increasing competition in a global economy, it is no wonder that U.S. employers are reducing or eliminating health coverage, if it was offered at all, for employees and retirees. The burden of ESI has become critical for U.S. auto manufacturers, as graphically illustrated by Figure 5.3, with overseas manufacturers in countries with some form of universal coverage having far smaller outlays for health care.[49] As employers increase cost-sharing with their employees, growing numbers of workers find ESI coverage unaffordable and of less value. Take-up rates whereby eligible employees of large retailers pay more to continue their insurance, have fallen from 83.8 percent to 67.3 percent in the last 8 years.[50]

Figure 5.3

Healthcare Costs Per Car

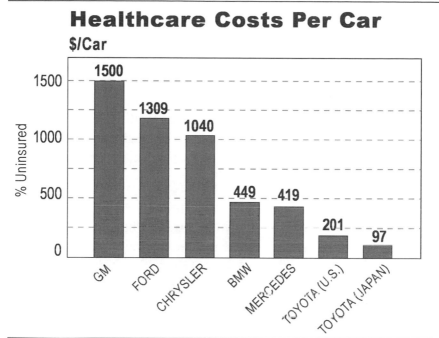

Source: *Modern Healthcare* Oct 24, 2005, 35(43):14. Applying the brakes. UAW deal to affect providers as well as workers.

The story is much the same in the individual market, where premiums (assuming people are accepted for coverage) are generally higher and benefits of less value than in the employer-based market. As noted earlier, the individual market is relatively small, involving only about 17 million non-elderly Americans. Individual coverage is difficult to obtain (or to keep). A 2006 study by the Commonwealth Fund found that 89 percent of Americans who explored getting individual coverage between 2003 and 2005 never purchased a plan.[51]

Elsewhere in the private market, the insurance industry also faces dimming prospects, except perhaps for short-term growth of near-useless LBP's. Insurers are finding it increasingly difficult to succeed in the Medigap market for supplemental coverage of Medicare recipients as seniors face more cost-sharing and growing out-of-pocket costs.[52] Because of high premiums, seniors with supplemental Medigap policies actually spend more on health care as a proportion of their income than any other group of seniors, including those without Medigap coverage.[53]

Association-based coverage is another part of the private market in sharp decline. Associations used to be a major source of health insurance for independent contractors and self-employed people, including many thousands in the professions, service, and entertainment sectors. As a result of premium increases and adverse selection, many association plans are disappearing. Ten years ago, one broker of association plans, Marsh Affinity Services, had 142 such clients. Today all but three have been closed down. At this writing more than 8,000 people with coverage through the California Association of Realtors will lose their coverage if Blue Shield of California is able to terminate the group's coverage.[54]

Factor 6: Subsidized Public Markets Are Also Vulnerable

As we saw in Chapter 1, health insurers have been shifting to privatized public programs in recent years as their prospects decline in traditional private markets. A recent *Wall Street Journal* editorial described the shift by large private insurers to the subsidized public market as the "new insurance frontier."[55] But even though they have found lucrative new markets in Medicare and Medicaid, these profits are likely to be short-lived as regulatory scrutiny increases and as legislators rein in subsidies. A brief summary of each program illustrates how attractive these markets have been to date, but also how vulnerable they are to future cutbacks.

The Medicare legislation of 2003 (MMA) has been a bonanza for the private sector, particularly for the insurance and drug industries. The MMA handed off the new prescription drug benefit for 42 million Medicare beneficiaries to these industries, with generous subsidies for each. Since the federal government was prohibited from negotiating bulk discounts for drugs and drug imports from Canada were banned, no price restraints were placed on drug manufacturers, which have responded by steadily increasing drug prices. Subsidies of about $46 billion over 10 years were allocated to private health plans (Medicare Advantage), in an effort to channel more Medicare patients into private plans.[56] By 2007, average overpayments to these plans was running about 112 percent of traditional FFS Medicare payments; private FFS plans were receiving 119 percent overpayments.[57] Prices were being stepped up at regular intervals throughout this private Medicare system.

Two examples show how profitable these privatized public programs can be for insurers. Premiums for the lowest-priced stand alone Part D prescription drug plans with doughnut-hole coverage increased by an average of 87 percent from 2006 to 2007.[58] Carl Martin, an analyst with CIBC World Markets in New York, had this to say about United Health Group's 22 percent gain in second-quarter 2007 profits from government-sponsored medical programs: "Medicare Advantage was a 'bright spot' for United Health in the quarter"... "This is likely a function of the benefit changes United Health made to its Medicare Advantage product this year, as it raised premiums, cut benefits and exited unprofitable counties."[59]

A backlash to industry profiteering is already underway. In the aftermath of the 2006 midterm elections, Democrats in Congress are attempting to level the playing field between private plans and FFS Medicare by cutting out subsidies and requiring private plans to compete on an equal basis with Medicare. Legislative efforts can also be expected to allow the government to negotiate drug prices.

Private insurers are countering that cutbacks of subsidies will not allow them to continue private plans, and we can anticipate that they will make good on this threat. Almost 10 years ago they did just that, when 2.4 million Medicare beneficiaries lost their private coverage as Medicare + Choice plans abandoned the market despite infusion of increased federal subsidies.[60,61]

Medicaid has also been a profitable market for private insurers, especially since 2000 as the employer-based insurance system continues to unravel. Medicaid gained 8 million new enrollees between 2000 and 2004 even as the ranks of the uninsured grew by 6 million.[62] Today the program covers about 55 million Americans, consuming one of every five dollars spent on U.S. health care. Medicaid accounts for the largest share of state budgets, and is growing by 8 percent a year.

Recognizing a new market, a number of investor-owned Medicaid HMOs jumped at their opportunity for growth, helped by conservative governors and legislators in a number of states who believe in market solutions to health care problems. The stock performance of the two leading Medicaid HMO companies (WellCare and Centene) have soared by 300 to 400 percent since their IPOs, all within the last 6 years. They are known on Wall Street as "pure plays." The top four new companies now manage the care of some 5 million Medicaid patients, and collect $9 billion in annual premiums. Amerigroup's revenues have gone up at an annual rate more than 60 percent over the last 10 years.[63]

This heyday for Medicaid HMOs is likely to be brief. Already they are facing litigation for abuses similar to those of private Medicare plans. A whistle-blower suit by a former Amerigroup employee in 2002, for example, led to a jury verdict by a Chicago court assessing $334 million in damages and civil penalties against both Amerigroup and its parent company. The company was found to be discriminating against pregnant women and other patients dubbed "unhealthies." Because of this cherry picking and weeding out of expensive patients, the company had an astoundingly profitable medical loss ratio. In 2002 and 2003, the ratios were below 50 percent. That is, more than 50 cents of every premium dollar went to administration and profits, not patient care. Judge Harry Leinenweber, who presided over the case, put it bluntly, writing that Amerigroup "pilfered money from Medicaid coffers to pad its own pockets." Amerigroup's CEO, Jeff McWaters, responded with a veiled threat "We've got some people trying to knock us down, but over time, they will stand down, because what we do is valid, capitalistic, and ethical." "But if profits do shrink, then how investors react will have a major impact on the Medicaid landscape."[64]

According to an analysis by *Fortune* magazine reporters, political connections and conflicts of interest are rife among Medicaid HMO companies. In Florida, for example, WellCare executives and their family members, together with the company PAC, contributed $1.5 million to Florida candidates for state and federal elections in 2006. In 2007, friendly Florida legislators slipped a rate increase into Florida's budget as they removed a state requirement that insurers spend at least 80 cents of each premium dollar on behavioral health services.[65]

Factor 7: Ineffective State and Federal Regulation
A short review of legislation reveals a great deal of effort with only limited results. Regulation of the private insurance industry has historically been the prerogative of the states. Over the years the federal government has largely supported the role of state insurance regulators, dating back to the McCarran-Ferguson Act of 1944, which stated that "the business of insurance shall be subject to the laws of the several states." [66]

Since the 1970s, however, the federal government has played an influential role on several occasions. The Employee Retirement Income Security Act of 1974 (ERISA) was intended to protect pension plans, but limited states' regulatory powers by exempting all self-funded employer health plans from state regulation. Large employers and insurers welcomed this legislation, and a new market opportunity was developed for organizations which could offer corporate health benefit programs on a multi-state or national basis.[67] By the late 1990s, it was estimated that more than one-third of the 150 million privately insured Americans were covered by such self-insured plans.[68]

The Consolidated Omnibus Reconciliation Act of 1985 (COBRA) was intended to help people who lose their jobs by requiring insurers and health plans to continue their previous coverage for at least 18 months. Two additional federal laws were passed in 1996 in an effort to protect consumers from various abuses by the insurance industry. The Health Insurance and Accountability Act (HIPAA) included provisions that discouraged insurers and HMOs from limiting or denying coverage for pre-existing conditions (for more than 12 months), required insurers and health plans to offer coverage to small employers with 2 to 50 employees, and required renewability of employer-based coverage as long as premiums were paid except in cases of fraud or misrepresentation by an employer.[69] The Mental Health Parity Act of 1998 (Domenici-Wellstone Bill) was enacted in an effort to establish some degree of parity with physical, biomedical disorders and to redress disparities and inequities in the provision of mental health services.[70]

The many kinds of abuses by private health insurers described in Chapter 3 have attracted the scrutiny of state regulators, and many states have passed legislation in attempts to improve access to health insurance, contain rising costs of insurance, and set standards for coverage. By the mid-1990s, 36 states had enacted guaranteed issue laws and 46 had passed guaranteed renewability laws for the small group market.[71] Ten states have passed regulations that all insurers use community rating or adjusted community rating for small group policies.[72] All states now require that some benefits be covered (egs., all 50 states require coverage for mammograms and well-child care while 27 require that cervical cancer screening be covered).[73]

Despite these efforts over many years by state and federal regulators, however, the private health insurance industry has been able to get around many of these attempted reforms. The private health insurance market is very complex, with three distinct parts—large group, small group, and individual— all of which vary by state. The market is thereby divided into 150 different state-level markets.

Insurers shop among states for the most favorable regulatory environment, and have found many creative ways to avoid regulation they consider onerous in each of these markets.[74] These examples make the point.

- When state regulators try to force employers to offer new mandated benefits, some employers escape to their self-insurance exemption under ERISA or drop coverage altogether.[75]
- A major loophole in HIPPA is the avoidance of regulating premium increases for policy renewals in the individual market[76]; an individual in one state was charged an increase of 2,000 percent after a change in health status.[77]
- Only one in four workers who lose their jobs can afford the premiums to continue coverage under COBRA.[78]
- When states attempt to improve access to mental health services, health plans that were providing such services may impose new restrictions (egs., cut coverage by visit time or days per year) or drop coverage entirely.[79]
- Health insurers can also circumvent state regulations by creating a group to which the insurer issues a master group policy, then selling individual certificates under the master policy, often across state lines.[80]

The insurance lobby has been extremely strong for many years in state houses across the country. As a nonprofit, nonpartisan research organization, the Washington D.C.-based Center for Public Integrity reported in 2002 that 2,269 insurance-related companies and organizations deployed a much larger number of lobbyists in the states. They lobby against regulatory intervention, typically citing the adverse impact of regulation which forces them to raise premiums and reduce coverage.[81] A 2005 analysis of state regulations by the conservative Heritage Foundation stated this clearly: "often overlooked is the fact that government policy, particularly excessive regulatory intervention, may price many Americans out of coverage and thus contribute to the high numbers of uninsured."[82] Moreover, many states balk at federal intrusion into their regulatory roles, and Congress has not appropriated sufficient funds for public education, oversight, and enforcement.[83]

Factor 8: Growing Economic Insecurity and Hardship, Even for the Insured

Adding to this ominous list of factors affecting the viability of private health insurance, from changes in employer support to flat wages of many Americans threatening to undercut their profitability, other important factors are in play.

Major demographic changes are underway in recent decades, which are rendering most middle class Americans, even if insured, vulnerable to catastrophic medical bills. Wages are stagnant for many working Americans, an increasing proportion of jobs pay poorly with meager benefits, and health insurance coverage is unstable, with turn-over often in three or four years. The gap between the affluent and poor has widened over the last 25 years, as shown in Figure 5.4, while U.S. household debt has soared to a record $11.4 trillion in 2005.[84] Since 2000, the number of Americans living at less than one-half of the federal poverty line has grown by 32 percent.[85] All of this has led Lance Dickie of the *Seattle Times* to this painful assessment:[86]

> *"Not long ago, the observation that unpaid medical bills are the No. 1 cause of personal bankruptcy might have been mildly interesting, like the unemployment rate if you have a steady job. Instead there is an unsettling recognition of vulnerability.*
>
> *The middle class watches as medical benefits are cut as they grow more expensive or are lost altogether. Parents worry about grown children going without insurance because of the cost or employers who do not provide it.*
>
> *Two short generations out from broad employer-based coverage grandchildren come into the world without the neonatal talisman of economic stability, a health-insurance card."*

The unaffordability of insurance and health care has become an economic and personal hardship. Figure 5.5 illustrates the extent

Figure 5.4

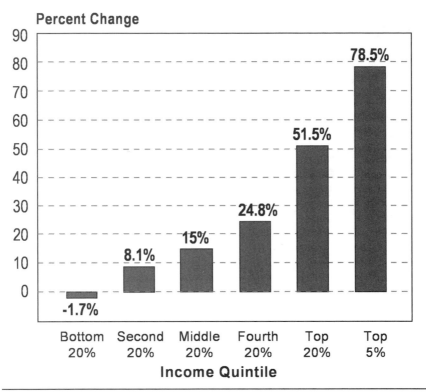

Change in Real Family Income, 1979-2004

Percent Change

Source: Bureau of the Census

of access problems for middle-class families with incomes between $25,000 and $50,000,[87] while Figure 5.6 shows how adults with chronic illness are faring with the costs of their care.[88] Almost 7 million Americans under age 65 who become disabled quickly lose employer-sponsored coverage, usually can't afford COBRA premiums because they are out of work, the premiums are high, and they also may face medical bills not covered by insurance. On top of these problems, they face a two-year waiting period before getting Medicare coverage; during this waiting period, 12 percent of them die.[89] One of every four families dealing with cancer is impoverished by that battle. For the insured, the odds aren't much better: one in five of insured families face poverty.[90] Two million Americans fall into bankruptcy each year as a result of medical bills, an increase of 2000 percent since 1981.[91] And bankruptcy filings are increasing rapidly—up 18 percent in the single month of January 2008 and up by 28 percent over a year earlier as a result of rising energy prices, the weakening housing market and soaring personal debts. [92]

As a result of surging costs of health care way beyond the means of most Americans, the impact on future generations appears dire. As an example, a recent 2008 report by the Center for Retirement Research at Boston College calculated the increasing proportions of Americans who will be "at risk" of being unable to maintain their standard of living in retirement. As Figure 5.7 shows, once health care costs are factored in, the percentage of households "at risk" in retirement rises to 61 percent overall and to more than two-thirds for generation Xers.[93]

Figure 5.5

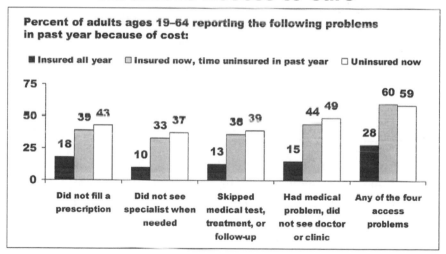

Lacking Health Insurance for Any Period Threatens Access to Care

Percent of adults ages 19–64 reporting the following problems in past year because of cost:

■ Insured all year   ▨ Insured now, time uninsured in past year   ☐ Uninsured now

Reprinted with permission from Collins S.R., Davis K., Doty M.M., Kriss J.L., & Holmgren A.L. Gaps in Health Insurance: An All-American Problem. Findings From the Commonwealth Fund Biennial Health Insurance Survey. The Commonwealth Fund, April 2006

There is still a widely held misconception that we have a functional safety net of programs which can help those confronting the perils of disease, injury, and disability. Unfortunately, this is no longer the case, if it ever was. As the principal safety net program, Medicaid

Figure 5.6

Adults Without Insurance are Less Likely to Be Able to Manage Chronic Conditions

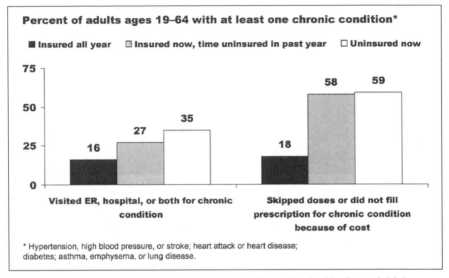

Percent of adults ages 19–64 with at least one chronic condition*

■ Insured all year   ▣ Insured now, time uninsured in past year   ☐ Uninsured now

Visited ER, hospital, or both for chronic condition

Skipped doses or did not fill prescription for chronic condition because of cost

* Hypertension, high blood pressure, or stroke; heart attack or heart disease; diabetes; asthma, emphysema, or lung disease.

Reprinted with permission from Collins S.R., Davis K., Doty M.M., Kriss J.L., & Holmgren A.L. Gaps in Health Insurance: An All-American Problem. Findings From the Commonwealth Fund Biennial Health Insurance Survey. The Commonwealth Fund, April 2006

is full of holes, with no relief on the horizon. A comprehensive 2007 report by Public Citizen's Health Research Group *Unsettling Scores: A Ranking of State Medicaid Programs*, describes just how porous this safety net has become. Many Americans fail to qualify for Medicaid coverage even with incomes below the federal poverty level and with illnesses that have rendered them poor. Many states impose severe restrictions on coverage, excluding such services as diagnostic, screening, and preventive services, rehabilitation services, private duty nursing services, medical devices and equipment. As Public Citizen's report notes "Lofty in its goals but often miserly in its actual impact on people, Medicaid mirrors changing economic circumstances, conflicting political pressures, and fluctuating demographic and medical needs."[94]

As if the above is not sufficiently bad news for our health care system and the 300 million Americans it is intended to serve, the future looks worse. Robert Reich, Professor of Public Policy at the Universi-

Figure 5.7

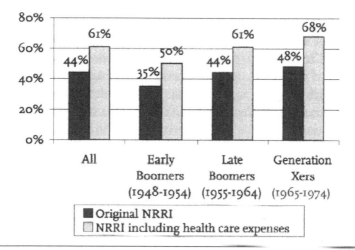

Effect of Health Care on the National Retirement Risk Index, 2006

Source: Munnell A. H., Soto M., Golub-Sass F., & Muldoon D. Health care costs drive up the national retirement risk index. Center for Retirement Research. Boston College, February 2008, no. 8-3. Reprinted with permission.

ty of California Berkeley and former Secretary of Labor in the Clinton Administration, sees us already in a recession. As a result of the one-two punch of the credit crunch and housing slump he observes: "Now several million Americans may lose their homes, and tens of millions more have only their credit cards to live on and are reaching the outer limits of what they can spend. As consumer spending shrinks, companies will reduce production and cut payrolls. That has already begun to happen. It's called recession."[95]

Jeremy Grantham, Chief Investment Strategist at Boston-based GMO and highly respected market analyst, views our current financial crisis as the worst in the post-war era. He notes that this crisis is more global than the savings-and-loan crisis, that economic hard times will not end soon, and that the trend-line value of the S & P in 2010 is 1100.[96] Recent press reports seem to confirm that this economic downturn will be severe and not easily reversed, as reflected by such signs as increasing home foreclosures, drop in housing starts, decline in consumer confidence and retail sales, falling industrial production, and turmoil in the banking and credit industries.[97-99]

Why We Must Discard Private
Multi-Payer Financing

The foregoing eight factors in the downhill course of the private health insurance industry not only portend its death knell but also show how ill-suited it is as a financing mechanism for U.S. health care. The 60-year report card for the industry is in, and it has failed the public interest. We now have an overgrown private insurance bureaucracy, the most expensive in the world, which resists reform or regulation and is pricing itself beyond the reach of middle-class America even as it offers "coverage" of less and less value. Table 5.1 lists the major reasons for the obsolescence of the industry in this country. Table 5.2 lists the top 5 implications for consumers of the downhill course of this industry.

TABLE 5.1

Why Private Health Insurance is Obsolete

- Inefficiencies vs public-financing
- Fragments risk pools by medical underwriting
- Increasing epidemic of underinsurance
- Excessive administrative and overhead costs
- Profiteering—shareholders trump patients
- Pricing itself out of the market
- Unsustainable and resists regulation

All this should come as no surprise. We have seen how market competition in the health care industry does not work to the advantage of the consumer, as it often does in other industries. The basic disconnect is that the business model serves corporate stakeholders and their investors as the first priority, not the needs of patients and their families. This does not mean that the insurance industry is evil, since that is only good business, but that we should have a financing system that puts patients first.

The death march of the industry has occurred even during mostly good economic times. As the odds of a serious recession grow,

Table 5.2

What the Dying Insurance Industry Means For Consumers

1. Continued escalation of uncontrolled costs of health care

2. Less insurance coverage for higher costs
- More cost-sharing
- Fewer benefits
- Unaffordable premiums
- Less continuity and reliability of coverage

3. More insecurity over access to health care
- More difficulty finding and keeping a primary care physician
- More bankruptcies due to medical bills
- Increasing inequities and disparities by income and race
- Worse health outcomes due to lack of access to necessary care

4. Continued decline of employer-sponsored insurance
- Increasing unaffordability of coverage in individual market

5. More corporate lobbying and disinformation as the industry fights a last-ditch battle for survival
- Increased political pressure to prop up the industry by tax breaks and subsidies (eg., overpayments to private Medicare plans)
- Increasing political activity by the industry, together with other corporate allies (egs., drug and medical device industries) in efforts to preserve deregulated health care markets
- Increased fraud and conflicts of interest within the industry and its relationship with government and regulatory agencies

we can only anticipate that the industry will become even more irrelevant to the needs of the public for affordable health care.

As the health care crisis builds in this country, our policy makers and legislators are still mostly in denial. A flurry of new state mandates is occurring across the country, all geared to promote wider use of private insurance while neglecting the fundamental reality that the private health insurance industry is failing due to growing problems. These efforts are flawed in targeting becoming insured as the policy goal without considering the affordability of health care itself. It does little good to "cover" people with low-cost limited-benefit policies when they can't afford and forego necessary health care. The insurance industry cannot make health care itself more affordable, as its track record shows. And if premiums are made more affordable, people with greater health care needs are excluded from coverage and more financial barriers are placed before individuals and families seeking care.

We obviously need a more effective way to pool risk and assure Americans equitable access to necessary health care. We will return to how best to replace the dying insurance industry in the last chapter. But for now we move to the next chapter to consider a wide range of incremental reform options that have been tried or are currently being proposed and ask whether any can achieve universal access to health care, not just insurance.

References

1. Bryan J.E. Blue Shield's role in the future of medicine. *Medical Economics* July 1954, as cited in Cunningham R, III, & Cunningham R.M. Jr. *The Blues: A History of the Blue Cross and Blue Shield System.* DeKalb, IL: Northern Illinois University Press, 1997, p 96.
2. Wolfson B. "Vicious cycle" of care. *The Orange County Register*, March 20, 2005.
3. Hacker J.S. *The Great Risk Shift: The Assault on American Jobs, Families, Health Care, and Retirement, and How You Can Fight Back.* New York: Oxford University Press, 2006, p 143.
4. Geyman J. P. *The Corrosion of Medicine: Can The Profession Reclaim Its Moral Legacy?* Monroe, ME: Common Courage Press, 2008.

5. Poisal J.A., Truffer C., Smith S., Sisko A, Cowan C., et al. and the National Health Expenditure Accounts Projections Team (Centers for Medicare and Medicaid Services) Health Spending Projections Through 2016. *Health Affairs Web Exclusive*, W242, February 21, 2007.

6. Keehan S. , Sisko A, et al. Center for Medicare and Medicaid Services. Office of the Actuary, National Health Statistics Group. Health Spending Projections Through 2017:The Baby-Boom Generation is Coming to Medicare. *Health Aff (Millwood)* February 26, 2008.

7. Nichols L.M., et al. Are market forces strong enough to deliver efficient health care systems? Confidence is waning. *Health Aff (Millwood)* 23(2):8-21, 2004.

8. Kronick R., Goodman D.C., Weinberg J., & Wagner E. The marketplace in health care reform. The demographic limitations of managed competition. *N Engl J Med* 328:148, 1993.

9. Associated Press, Study: health insurers are near monopolies. April 18, 2006.

10. Nyman J.A. Is "moral hazard" inefficient? The policy implications of a new theory. *Health Aff (Millwood)* 23(5):194-99, 2004.

11. Davis K. *Half of Insured Adults with High-Deductible Health Plans Experience Medical Bill or Debt Problems*. New York, Commonwealth Fund, January 27, 2005.

12. Artiga S. & O"Malley M. Increasing premiums and cost sharing in Medicaid and SCHIP: Recent state experiences. Issue Paper. Kaiser Commission on Medicaid and the Uninsured. Kaiser Family Foundation, May 2005, p 2.

13. Preker A.S. The introduction of universal access to health care in the OECD: Lessons for developing countries. In: *Achieving Universal Coverage of Health Care*, Nitagyarumphong E.S. & Mills A. (editors) Ministry of Public Health, Bangkok, 1998, p 103.

14. Kaiser Family Foundation. Report #7527. Employer Health Benefits: 2006 Summary of Findings, Menlo Park, Calif, 2006.

15. Barry P. & Basler B. Healing our system. *AARP Bulletin*, 48(3):March 2007, p2.

16. Johnston D.C. "05 incomes, on average, still below 2000 peak. *New York Times*, August 21, 2007:C1.

17. Schoen C., How S.K.H., Weinbaum I., Craig J.E. & Davis K. Public views on shaping the future of the U.S. health system. New York: The Commonwealth Fund, 2006.

18. *Consumer Reports*. Are you really covered? Why 4 in 10 Americans can't depend on their health insurance. September 2007. http://www.consumerreports.org/cro/index.htm.

19. Patchias E. M.,& Waxman J. Women and health coverage. The affordability gap. Issue Brief. New York: The Commonwealth Fund, April 2007.

20. Pollitz K., Koffman M., Salganicoff A. & Ranji U. Maternity care and consumer-driven health plans. Henry J. Kaiser Family Foundation. Washington, D.C., June 2007.

21. Henderson N. Greenspan's mixed legacy: America prospered during the Fed chiefs tenure, but built up massive debt. *Washington Post National Weekly Edition.* January 30, February 5, 2006, p 6.

22. Washington Post. Household credit card debt. *Washington Post National Weekly Edition.* June 4-10, 2007, p 24.

23. Ip G. Not your father's pay: Why wages today are weaker. *Wall Street Journal*, May 25, 2007, A2.

24. Price Waterhouse Coopers Health Research Institute. Behind the numbers: Healthcare cost trends for 2008, June 20, 2007.

25. Hewitt Associates. HMOs will seek 14.1 percent increase in premiums by 2008, as cited in Kaiser Daily Health Policy Report, July 3, 2007.

26. U.P.I.Economist bashes Bush HSA proposal. United Press International, February 6, 2006.

27. Graham Center One-Pager. Who will have health insurance in 2025? *Am Fam Physician* 72(10):1989, 2005.

28. American Diabetes Association. Gaps found in all components of private health insurance coverage for people with diabetes. Alexandria, VA: February 8, 2005.

29. Kaiser Family Foundation. Survey of Families Affected by Cancer Shows People With and Without Health Insurance Often Suffer Serious Financial Hardships. *USA Today*/Kaiser Family Foundation/Harvard School of Public Health National Survey of Households Affected by Cancer. November 20, 2006.

30. Families USA. Special report. Coverage through the "doughnut hole" grows scarier in 2007. November 2006.

31. Appleby J. Is a little medical coverage that much better than none? *USA Today*, June 6, 2007, 1A.

32. Gabel J, Pickreign J, McDevitt R, Whitmore II, Gandolfo L, et al. Trends in the Golden State: Small-Group Premiums Rise Sharply While Actuarial Values for Individual Coverage Plummet. *Health Affairs Web Exclusive*, June 14, 2007.

33. Schoen C., Doty M., Collins S.R., & Holmgren A.L. Commonwealth Fund,

Insured but not protected: How many adults are underinsured, the experiences of adults with inadequate coverage mirror those of their uninsured peers, especially among the chronically ill. *Health Affairs Web Exclusive*, June 14, 2005.

34. Blumberg L. J., Holahan J., Hadley J., & Norclah K. Setting a standard of affordability for health insurance coverage. *Health Affairs Web Exclusive*, June 4, 2007.

35. Maxwell S, et al. Growth in Medicare and out-of-pocket spending: Impact on vulnerable beneficiaries. New York: The Commonwealth Fund, 2000.

36. Blumenthal D, et al. *Renewing the Promise: Medicare & Its Reform.* New York: Oxford University Press, 1988, p 26.

37. Neuman P., Cubanski J., Desmond KA., & Rice T. H. How much "skin in the game" do Medicare beneficiaries have? The increasing financial burden of health care spending, 1997-2003. *Health Aff* 26(6): 1692-1701, 2007.

38. Families USA. Too great a burden: America's families at risk. December 2007.

39. Geymun J. P. *Falling Through The Safety Net: Americans Without Health Insurance,* Monroe, ME: Common Courage Press, 2004.

40. Krugman P. The world of U.S. health care economics is downright scary. *Seattle Post Intelligencer*, September 26, 2006:B1.

41. Grembowski D.E., Diehr P., Novak L.C., Roussel A.F., & Morton D.P. Measuring the "managedness" and covered benefits of health plans. *Health Services Research*, 35(3):707, 2000.

42. Kagel R. Blue crossroads: Insurance in the 21ˢᵗ Century. *American Medical News*, September 20, 2004.

43. Krugman P. Passing the buck. *New York Times*, April 22, 2005.

44. Silber J. Kaiser adds deductibles to some insurance plans. *Contra Costa Times*, April 29, 2004.

45. Colliver V. Retiree Health Benefits Decline. *San Francisco Chronicle*, December 15, 2004, C1.

46. Freudenheim M. Fewer Employers Totally Cover Health Premiums. *New York Times*, March 23, 2005.

47. U.S. Census. Kaiser Foundation. Changes in Employees' Health Insurance Coverage, 2001-2005, October 2006.

48. Holahan J., & Cook A. Why did the number of uninsured continue to increase in 2005? Issue paper #7571. Kaiser Commission on Medicaid and the Uninsured. Kaiser Family Foundation, October 2006.

49. Taylor M. Applying the brakes: UAW deal to affect providers as well as workers (United Auto Workers union). *Modern Health Care* 35(43):October 24, 2005, p 14.

50. Fuhrmans V. Citing cost concerns, more workers leave firms' health plans. *Wall Street Journal*, August 25, 2006:A9.

51. Collins S., et al. Squeezed: Why rising exposure to health care costs threatens the health and financial well-being of American families. Commonwealth Fund, September 2006.

52. Hacker J.S. Privatizing risk without privatizing the welfare state: The hidden politics of social policy retrenchment in the United States. *American Political Science Review* 98, no. 2 May 2004, 253.

53. Desmond K.A., Rice T., Cubanski J., & Newman P. The Burden of Out-of-Pocket Health Spending Among Older Versus Younger Adults: Analysis from the Consumer Expenditure Survey, 1998-2003. The Henry J. Kaiser Family Foundation, September 2007.

54. Girion L. Health insurance options dwindle for self-employed. Group plans are being dropped or becoming unaffordable to many. *Los Angeles Times*, March 27, 2007.

55. Editorial. The new insurance frontier. *Wall Street Journal*, January 7, 2007: A12.

56. Geyman J.P. *Shredding the Social Contract: The Privatization of Medicare.* Monroe, Me: Common Courage Press, 2006, pp 59-62.

57. Medicare Rights Center. Medicare private plan overpayments: No bang for the buck. *Asclepios* 7 (21), May 24, 2007.

58. Gerencher K. States with insurance holes in Medicare drug plans on rise. *Wall Street Journal*, November 8, 2006:D7.

59. Goldstein A. United Health profit rises on government-sponsored medical programs. Bloomberg.com, July 19, 2007.

60. CMS Medicare Fact Sheet. Centers for Medicare and Medicaid Services, September 2002.

61. Waldholz M. Prescriptions. Medicare seniors face confusion as HMOs bail out of program. *Wall Street Journal*, D4, October 3, 2002.

62. Krugman P., & Wells R. The health care crisis and what to do about it. *The New York Review of Books* 53(5), March 23, 2006.

63. McLean B. The big money in Medicaid: A boom in HMOs for the neediest leads to litigation, controversy—and lots of profits. *Fortune* 155(12):97-102, June 25, 2007.

64. Ibid #55, pp 100, 102.

65. Ibid #55, p 102.

66. 15 U.S.C. section 1012, as cited in Kofman M. & Pollitz K. Health insurance regulation by states and the federal government: A review of current approaches and proposals for change. Washington, D.C., Health Policy Institute, Georgetown University, April 2006.

67. Gray B. H. The rise and decline of the HMO: A chapter in U.S. health policy. In: Stevens R.A., Rosenberg C.E., & Burns L.R. *History and health policy in the United States: Putting the past back in.* New Brunswick, NJ: Rutkers University Press, 2006, p325.

68. Noble A., & Brennan TA. The States of Managed-Care Regulation: Developing Better Rules. In: *The Challenge of Regulating Managed Care,* eds. Billi J., & Agrawal G.B. Ann Arbor: University of Michigan Press, 2001, pp 29-57.

69. Atchinson B.S., & Fox D. M. The politics of the Health Insurance Portability and Accountability Act. *Health Aff (Millwood)* 16(3):146-50, 1997.

70. Frank R.G., Koyanagi C., & McGuire T.G. The politics and economics of mental health "parity" laws. *Health Aff (Millwood)* 16(4):108-19, 1997.

71. Blue Cross Blue Shield Report. State Legislative Health Care and Insurance Issues: 2005 Survey of Plans, December 2005, p 57.

72. Kofman R., & Pollitz K. Health insurance regulation by states and the federal government. A review of current approaches and proposals for change. Washington, D.C., Health Policy Institute, Georgetown University, April 2006.

73. Ibid #71, p 74.

74. Hall M. The geography of health insurance regulation: A guide to identifying, exploiting, and policing market boundaries. *Health Aff (Millwood)* 19(2):173-82, 2000.

75. Kleinke J.D. *Oxymorons: The myths of the U.S. health care system.* San Francisco: Jossey-Bass, 2001, p 189.

76. Patel V. & Pauly M.V. Guaranteed renewability and the problem of risk variation in individual health insurance markets. *Health Affairs Web Exclusive,* August 28, 2002, p W284.

77. Pollitz K., Tapay N., Hadley E., & Specht J. Early experience with "new federalism" in health insurance regulation. *Health Aff (Millwood)* 19(4):7-22, 2000.

78. Commonwealth Fund. Only one-fourth of workers would keep health coverage through COBRA if they lost their jobs. Press release. August 29, 2002.

79. Frank R.G., Kovanagi C., & McGuire T.G. The politics and economics of mental health "parity" laws. *Health Aff (Millwood)* 16(4):108, 1997.

80. Ibid #74.

81. Renzulli D. and the Center for Public Integrity. *Capitol Offenders: How Private Internists Govern Our States*. Washington, D.C., Public Integrity Books, 2002, p 95.

82. New M.J. The effect of state regulations on health insurance premiums: A preliminary analysis. Center for Data Analysis Report #05-07. The Heritage Foundation, October 27, 2005.

83. Ibid #77, p. 7.

84. Ibid #21.

85. U.S. Census Bureau, as cited in Harper's Index, *Harper's* 314 (885):June 2007, p 33.

86. Dickie L. Winds of change carrying cries for health care toward the ill. *Seattle Times*, March 23, 2007.

87. Kaiser Family Foundation, NPR/Kaiser Survey, June 2002.

88. Collins S.R., Davis K., Doty M.M., Kriss J. L., & Holmgren A.L. Gaps in health insurance: An All-American problem. The Commonwealth Fund, April 2006.

89. Medicare Rights Center. *Too Sick to Work, Too Soon for Medicare: The Human Cost of the Two-Year Medicare Waiting Period for Americans with Disabilities.http://www.medicarerights.org/*Too_Sick to_Work_Too Soon for_Medicare. pdf.

90. Sack K. Cancer Society Focuses Its Ads on the Uninsured. *The New York Times*, August 31, 2007.

91. Himmelstein D. U., Warren E., Thorne D. & Woolhandler S. Illness and injury as contributors to bankruptcy. *Health Affairs Web Exclusive* W5-63, 2005.

92. Anderson J. Filings for bankruptcy up 18 percent in January. *New York Times*, March 5, 2008:C3.

93. Munnell A. H., Soto M., Webb A., Golub-Sass F., & Muldoon D. Health care costs drive up the national retirement risk index. Center for Retirement Research. Boston College, February 2008, no. 8-3.

94. Ramirez de Arrelano A.B. & Wolfe S. M. Unsettling Scores: A Ranking of State Medicaid Programs. Washington, D.C. Public Citizen Health Research Group, April 2007.

95. Reich R. The politics of an economic nightmare. *The Progressive Populist* 14(4):March 1, 2008, p 12.

96. Ward S. This credit crisis has a long way to run. Interview with Jeremy Grantham, Chief Investment Strategist, GMO *Barron's* February 11, 2008.

97. Goodman, P S, Economic squeeze moves from Wall St. to Main St. *New York Times*, March 21, 2008: A1

98. Davis, B, Ip, G, Paletta, D, U. S. mulls next steps in crisis. *Wall Street Journal*, March 18, 2008: A1

99. Corkery, M, Mortgage mess hits home for nation's small builders. *Wall Street Journal,* March 21, 2008: A1

CHAPTER 6

Saving Lives or Saving the Industry?: Why Incremental System "Reforms" Continue to Fail

"The only thing new in the world is the history you don't know."
—President Harry Truman[1]

"Medical history teaches us where we come from, where we stand in medicine at the present time, and in what direction we are marching. It is the compass that guides us into the future."
—Henry E. Sigerist (1891-1957)
Leading medical historian and former Professor
and Director of the Institute of the History of Medicine
at Johns Hopkins University[2]

As we have seen in earlier chapters, problems of decreasing access, uncontrolled costs, uneven quality, disparities and inequities increasingly plague U.S. health care as health care services become ever more unaffordable for growing parts of the population. With private health insurance on its death bed, the proposed cures are being bandied about louder than ever. Where are they taking us?

Many incremental attempts have been made to address these problems over the years. They have tinkered around the margins of the marketplace, leaving in place the private health insurance industry with wide latitude to continue its quest to preserve profits while avoiding coverage of sicker Americans. As we will soon see, all of the "reforms" that have been implemented buttress rather than solve the core problem: private health insurance doesn't work.

Two major incremental reform efforts have attempted to prop up employer-sponsored coverage or encourage wider use of individual insurance coverage, as illustrated by the "consumer-directed" health care movement and individual mandates. All of these efforts have failed to remedy growing system problems. Market advocates are now promoting a variety of other incremental approaches, such as expanded use of chronic disease management and information technology, as fixes to system problems without recognizing the ongoing failure of any of these incremental efforts. In effect then, health policy is proceeding apace, free of any understanding of a long history of failures and unencumbered by any evidence of what is actually needed.

This chapter undertakes three goals: (1) to briefly describe the experience of incremental reform attempts of the health care system; (2) to consider some major reasons why these attempts fail to remedy system problems; and (3) to discuss where we can go from here to reform health care.

What Has Been Tried?

Before considering the effects of incremental efforts to reform the U.S. health care system, we need to summarize its major problems. Table 6.1 lists what seem to me to be the most important macro-problems against which to measure the results of reform attempts. Admittedly, our market-based non-system is very fragmented and complex. Some would argue with this list, perhaps deleting some problems and adding others. But most would probably agree that increasing costs and decreasing access trump, and often contribute to, the others.

Further, most of these problems are driven by multiple factors. For example, increasing costs have many drivers. These are the top nine, in my view:

1. Technology advances with "medical arms race" among facilities
2. Inappropriate and unnecessary care
3. Profiteering by providers, and by investor-owned companies and facilities
4. Aging of population
5. Increase in chronic disease
6. Expanding definitions of "disease"
7. Inefficiency and redundancy of 1,300 private insurers
8. Consumer demand with imprudent choices (moral hazard)
9. Defensive medicine due to medicolegal liability

Table 6.1

Major Problems of U.S. Health Care

1. Uncontrolled inflation of health care costs and prices

2. Growing crisis in unaffordability of health care now extending to middle class

3. Decreasing access to care

4. Increasing health disparities

5. Rising rates of uninsured and underinsured

6. Discontinuity and turnover of insurance coverage

7. Variable, often poor quality of care

8. High rates of inappropriate and unnecessary care with physician induced demand

9. Administrative complexity, profiteering and waste of 1,300 private insurers

10. Decreased choice of hospital and physician in managed care programs

11. Erosion of safety net programs

12. Declining primary care base

13. Inadequate national system for assessment of new medical technologies, insufficient use of cost-effectiveness analysis

14. Lax federal regulation of drug, medical device, and dietary supplement industries

15. Market-based system more accountable to stakeholders and investors than to patients

Again, others may disagree with this list, especially the lower priorities given to consumer demand and defensive medicine, but a rough sense of relative priorities is useful. We are already finding that the increased use of cost-sharing with patients under CDHC typically leads to underuse of necessary care, rather than control of imprudent discretionary care, the stated justification.[3-6] High levels of physician-induced demand are arguably a much more important cause of inflating health care costs than consumer demand, as illustrated by regional variation studies with estimates that up to one third of all health care services in the U.S. are either unnecessary or of little value.[7] The annual direct costs of malpractice litigation are estimated to be about $7 billion, while estimates of the indirect costs of defensive medicine range between $20 and $80 billion. These are huge figures, but at most they account for no more than about 4 percent of our $2.2 trillion health care bill.[8] While significant, these costs pale in comparison with the 31 percent of the health care dollar going to administrative expenses (mostly to our private health insurance industry)[9] or the 2006 assessment by the Centers for Medicare and Medicaid Services (CMS) that much of our accelerating health care costs are driven by new medical treatments, rising prices, and increased utilization of health care services.[10]

Building on Employer-Sponsored Health Insurance

As we saw in Chapter 1, employer-sponsored insurance (ESI) grew rapidly during and after the World War II years, aided by favorable tax policies with exemptions for both employers and employees of the costs of coverage. But over the last 60 years, the nation's economy and work force have changed dramatically, and the employer based system has continued to unravel. Faced with continued escalation of health care costs, employers as well as workers have found it increasingly difficult to afford the costs of health insurance.

Employers in 2008 are spending on average more than $9,300 per employee for health benefits.[11] Employers are now shifting more costs to employees on a defined contribution basis without the more comprehensive coverage of past policies. By 2006, the average annual premiums for employer-sponsored insurance (ESI) had risen to $4,242 for single coverage and $11,480 for a family of four.

According to the 2007 U.S. Census Bureau Report, there are now more uninsured (47 million) than at any time since passage of Medicare and Medicaid in 1965. The number of uninsured Americans increased by 2.18 million in 2006, the largest jump since 1992, with 93 percent of that increase among middle-and high-income families.[12] Only three of five employers now offer any coverage.[13]

Figure 6.1 shows marked changes in types of employer-based health plans since 1988, with the near-disappearance of conventional

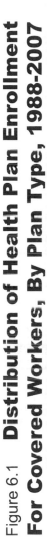

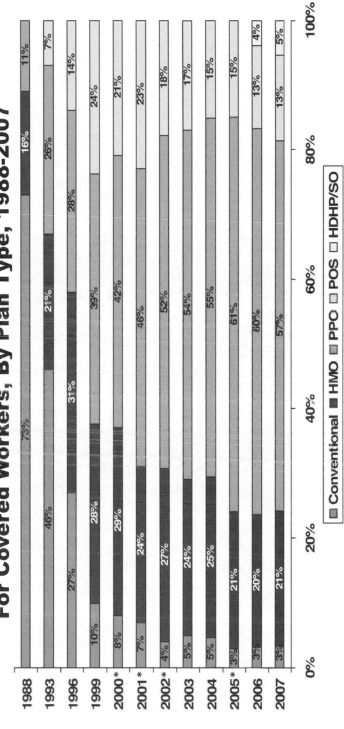

Figure 6.1 **Distribution of Health Plan Enrollment For Covered Workers, By Plan Type, 1988-2007**

*Distribution is statistically different from distribution for the previous year shown at p<.05. No statistical tests are conducted for year prior to 1999. No statistical tests are conducted between 2005 and 2005 due to the addition of HDHP/SO as a new plan type.

Source: Employer Health Benefits 2007 Annual Survey (#7672), The Henry J. Kaiser Family Foundation & HRET, September 2007. Reprinted with permission from the Henry J. Kaiser Family Foundation. The Kaiser Family Foundation, based in Menlo Park, California, is a non-profit, private operating foundation focusing on the major health care issues facing the nation and is not associated with Kaiser Permanente or Kaiser Industries.

plans and the rapid growth of PPOs.[14] More than one-half of small-business owners no longer offer their employees either health insurance or subsidies toward purchasing coverage, according to a recent poll by the National Federation of Independent Business (NFIB).[15] The demise of ESI was further accelerated by a recent policy decision by the Equal Employment Opportunity Commission that employers can reduce or eliminate health benefits for retirees when they reach 65 years of age and become eligible for Medicare.[16]

With a goal to increase the number of people covered by ESI, employer mandates (whereby employers are required to provide health insurance for their employees) have been tried for more than 30 years. President Nixon proposed such a plan ("play or pay") in the early 1970s, but Watergate and the Vietnam War diverted attention from health care and it was never enacted into law.[17] The State of Hawaii has had a 30-year experience with employer mandate; although it initially dropped the uninsured rate below 5 percent, that rate has since grown and the program has failed to control costs or avoid large increases in insurance premiums.[18] Employer mandates of various types were attempted by Massachusetts in 1988 and by Minnesota, Tennessee and Vermont in 1992 and 1993, but none were successful in reducing the number of uninsured.[19]

Many states are still experimenting with various kinds of employer mandates, including California, Connecticut, Massachusetts, Maine, Minnesota, New Mexico, Oregon, Vermont, and Wisconsin.[20] Some of these plans are combined with individual mandates, as in Massachusetts and California. They are generally opposed by the business community, Chambers of Commerce, and conservative market advocates.

Although touted by many proponents as the "Massachusetts Miracle" and a national model, the 2006 Massachusetts reform attempt illustrates some of the inherent problems of this approach. Two years later, it is still controversial and very much a work in progress, with no chance to provide universal coverage for all state residents, higher than expected costs of insurance, and serious concerns within the business community. Small businesses employ about two-thirds of the uninsured work force in Massachusetts. These employers fear their future cost burden for individual mandate coverage, with fines levied by the State for failing to make a "fair and reasonable" contribution to the costs of that coverage. These mandates depend upon the private insurance industry to provide expanded coverage, but even in a state that regulates the industry more than most other states, affordability of premiums still poses a big challenge for many lower-income workers. The plan includes no credible cost containment mechanisms and provides insufficient funding for promised subsidies.[21-22]

The failure of the "Massachusetts Miracle" has recently been described in these terms by Steffie Woolhandler and David Himmelstein, general internists and health policy experts at Harvard Medical School:[23]

"While the middle class sinks, the health reform law has buoyed our state's wealthiest health institutions. Hospitals like Massachusetts General are reporting record profits and enjoying rate increases tucked into the reform package. Blue Cross and other insurers that lobbied hard for the law stand to gain billions from the reform, which shrinks their contribution to the state's free care pool and will force hundreds of thousands to purchase their defective products. Meanwhile, new rules for the free care pool will drastically cut funding for the hundreds of thousands who remain uninsured, and for the safety-net hospitals and clinics that care for them. (Disclosure: We've practiced for the past 25 years at a public hospital that is currently undergoing massive budget cuts.)"

Employer mandates pose big problems for business. To the extent that they are a mandatory additional cost to business, they become an incentive to move out of state, to states that don't impose these mandates. Thus mandates are anti-business as well as of no value to the consumer. This raises a question: would the alternative single-payer insurance system where the government insures everyone be anti-business? This is an important question to which we will return in a later chapter.

CDHC and Individual Mandates

The consumer-choice model for health reform, as we have seen, is currently popular among many conservative and moderate legislators, business interests, and other policy makers for one simple reason. As the theory goes, by giving consumers more choices, they have "more skin in the game" to be prudent, becoming a force for containing health care costs. Consumer-directed health plans typically involve high-deductibles, co-payments, and other cost-sharing restrictions. They are often combined with either a health savings account (HSA) or health reimbursement arrangement (HRA). They may be offered by employers or otherwise promoted through the individual market, with such "enabling" strategies as tax credits and other subsidies to help people to afford insurance premiums.

Although CDHC is touted by its advocates as offering more choice and autonomy in the medical marketplace, it has been very slow to catch on. According to annual surveys by the Kaiser Family Foundation, only about 4 percent (2.7 million) of the 70 million American workers with ESI were enrolled in a high-deductible health plan with HSA in 2006, the same percentage as in 2005. Four in ten employees were offered no choice of other plans while only 19 percent of employees chose a CDHP over other options.[24]

HSAs are more likely to be taken up by healthy and more affluent people as a tax-sheltered investment device. A 2008 article in the *Wall Street Journal* hailed the tax advantages of HSAs as investment vehicles, noting that Merrill Lynch is managing about 20,000 HSAs for clients, mostly physicians, lawyers, and accountants.[25] Older and sicker people usually find them unaffordable and insufficient in their coverage.[26]

High deductible health plans (HDHPs), with higher cost-sharing with enrollees, lead many patients to delay or avoid necessary care for the simple reason that they increase out of pocket costs and encourage a wait and see attitude to health problems. They contribute to the growing trend of underinsurance, and often result in less preventive care, worse outcomes from later diagnosis, and higher costs of more complicated illness later on.[27] Moreover, they have no track record or promise of containing health care costs.[28] This is all the more clear since one-half of people with health insurance account for less than 5 percent of total annual health care expenditures, a consistent figure over many decades.[29]

CDHC and HSAs provide insurers and investment firms with yet another potential bonanza as they compete for an estimated $1 billion in annual fees for managing HSAs. United Health and Blue Cross have chartered their own banks and established special credit cards to manage these accounts.[30] Concerning the potential role of CDHC in health care reform, Himmelstein and Woolhandler draw this conclusion:[31]

"Behind the rhetoric of consumer responsiveness and personal responsibility, CDHC sets in motion huge resource transfers. The sick and middle-aged pay more, whereas the young and healthy pay less. Women spend more, whereas men spend less. Workers bear more of the burden, whereas employers bear less. The poor skip vital care while the rich enjoy tax-free tummy tucks. And, as in every health reform in memory, bureaucrats and insurance firms walk off with an ever larger share of health dollars."

Four states are now experimenting with individual mandates (California, Massachusetts, Oregon, and Pennsylvania), with other states watching their experience with interest.[32] States thereby require, under penalty for non-compliance, all uninsured state residents to purchase their own health insurance, with state subsidies for those who can't afford coverage. That places the affordability question front and center, as well as what income levels state legislators will define for subsidies.

There is still no widely accepted definition of affordability, and a 2006 study of Massachusetts' experience so far makes clear that out-of-pocket costs must be considered as well as costs of insurance premiums. This study found that median health spending of individuals and families across all incomes with non-group coverage was 16.9 percent and 14.7 percent of income, respectively, on health insurance and out-of-pocket costs. For ESI group coverage, those figures were 12.3 percent and 15.1 percent for individual and family coverage, respectively. Total medical spending, of course, can be very high for those with high medical needs and especially high as a percentage of total income for those with incomes below 300 percent of poverty.[33]

The Commonwealth Health Insurance Connector Authority in Massachusetts, charged with the task of implementing the individual mandate, has already found that it has had to exempt many more people from the mandate than anticipated after finding that the lowest cost private plans were unaffordable. Especially hard-hit are uninsured people between 50 and 64 years of age, who face very high insurance premiums for limited coverage, if they can so qualify. A recent report found that premiums for an unsubsidized plan for a 60 year-old are twice those for a 27-year old. Massachusetts AARP and a coalition of other organizations are pushing for expanded criteria to waive the mandate for this age group.[34]

The Connector Authority is still struggling with the definition of affordability and who needs subsidies.[35] This outcome is hardly surprising. Dr. Don McCanne sums up the dilemma this way:[36]

> *"Insisting that the program must be administered through private plans, the architects tinkered with the policies behind the concept. They gave up on enacting standard comprehensive benefits for everyone, and established four levels of coverage: bronze, silver, gold, and young adult. Since the less expensive plans were still unaffordable for many, they tinkered with numbers that would excuse many from the penalty that would be assessed for not buying the insurance that they could not afford. But in trying to come up with reasonable numbers, it turns out that a great many more will have to be excused from the penalty. Thus their universal program is not universal, and it will be even less so as the health care financing crisis deteriorates further."*

Other Incremental Reform Attempts

The following six strategies are the major ones put forward to incrementally reform our health care system. The first four are intended to increase the ranks of the insured, while the others target one or another aspect of cost, quality, and efficiency.

1. Tax Credits

Tax credits or vouchers have been promoted for many years by conservative policy makers as ways to enable uninsured people to better afford health insurance. They have long been a part of AMA policy and are also supported by other professional organizations and AHIP. A typical tax credit would provide low-income individuals with $1,000 reimbursement ($2,000 for families). But these amounts are far too small to help the uninsured to afford today's average health insurance premiums (more than $4,000 for single coverage and $11,000 for families of four). Tax credits discriminate against older and sicker individuals, and are ineffective in reducing the ranks of the uninsured. A recent RAND study found that government subsidies which cut health insurance premium costs by one-half would reduce the number of uninsured by only 3 percent.[37] MIT economist Jonathan Gruber concludes that tax policies involving private insurance are much less efficient than policies which expand public coverage.[38]

2. State High-Risk Pools

In hopes of increasing insurance opportunities for people denied coverage in the individual market, state high-risk pools have been established in 30 states with support of federal and state funding. However, they cover only about 180,000 people nationwide, and are largely ineffective. These high-risk pools are beset by many problems, including extended waiting lists, limited benefits (egs., exclusions of maternity care and mental health), high premiums, and limited state and federal budgets.[39] With one of the largest high-risk pools in the country, California covers only 0.0013 percent of its uninsured population in this way.[40]

3. Association Health Plans (AHPs)

Another approach favored by the insurance industry and conservative policy makers is the establishment of association health plans (AHPs). These are often set up by insurers as not-for-profit false fronts for their own for-profit marketing. In most states, AHPs are exempt from state rate-setting regulations. A comprehensive report on AHPs by Families USA in 2005 found widespread evidence of bait and switch premium hikes, misrepresentation of benefits, excessive cost-sharing with enrollees, and other evidence of fraud and abuse.[41] One typical scam was a 76 percent premium increase for thousands of families at the time of annual renewal.[42] Moreover, AHPs fail to contain costs and the Congressional Budget Office (CBO) has reported that most small employers experience increased costs.[43]

4. Chronic Disease Management

Since chronic illness accounts for almost 75 percent of annual health care expenditures,[44] it has attracted attention as a target for cost containment. Better management of chronic disease has long been a goal of integrated systems of care such as Kaiser Permanente and Group

Health Cooperative of Puget Sound. These institutions have pioneered in the development of new approaches to care based upon the Chronic Care Model, including electronic disease registries, evidence-based practice guidelines, support of patient self-management, and consultation with expert teams of physician and nurse specialists. [45,46]

A new, largely investor-owned industry has been developed by the drug industry, especially by pharmacy-benefit management companies (PBMs), since the early 1990s. Commercial disease management (DM) programs are designed to identify high-risk patients through claims data for selected chronic diseases, then sell programs of patient education and self-management to employers and managed care organizations. These programs are marketed as strategies to control costs and increase quality, but they serve their own interests by promoting their product lines and increasing sales. As with HSAs, a new large and lucrative market has opened up. As an example, Medco, as one of the country's three largest PBMs with revenues in 2006 of over $42 billion, purchased diabetes product supplies Poly Media Corporation in 2007 as a way to gain market share for the care of diabetes and obesity. [47]

Despite marketing hype by industry and the interest of employers and some managed care organizations, commercial DM programs, disconnected as they typically are from primary care, have yet to show any sustained impact on cost containment or quality of care.[48] The CBO reported in 2004 that "there is insufficient evidence to conclude that disease management programs can generally reduce overall health spending..."[49] A recent analysis by Rand of 317 studies of disease management programs for various diseases concluded that, while the process of care can be improved for some conditions, there is little evidence that these programs can actually save money or improve health outcomes over the long term. The Rand study further advised that "payers and policy makers should remain skeptical about vendor claims and should demand supporting evidence based on transparent and scientifically sound methods."[50]

5. Pay-for-Performance (P4P)

P4P initiatives are taking place over the last several years among some health plans and as a demonstration project within the Medicare program. While they may appear to some to be reasonable approaches to encourage improved quality of care, their track record so far is not impressive and there are many problems with the process and concept. A three-year national study of a P4P pilot program involving treatment guidelines for more than 100,000 Medicare patients with acute myocardial infarction found no incremental improvement in quality of care or outcomes in 54 study hospitals compared to 446 control hospitals.[51] The Community Tracking Study has identified one or another P4P program underway in all 12 communities being tracked. There is little consensus or standardization of performance measures, however, due to preferences and resistance of providers and local market conditions.[52]

A giant new industry has been created which mines aggregated electronic claims data (without patients' names), then attempts to profile physicians by cost efficiency and/or quality of care. In the Washington, D.C. metropolitan area, for example, United Health Care has launched a Web site ranking physicians with zero, one, or two stars. Since claims data are the easiest to collect, they are being adopted by many payers as a means to develop tiered provider networks, typically more on the basis of "cost efficiency" than for quality.

There are many problems, however, with the credibility of claims data for these purposes. Claims data cannot reflect clinical outcomes, the preferred standard of quality assessment. Criteria for profiling lack standardization and vary widely from one payer to another. Some physicians may be rated in the top tier by one payer and the bottom tier by another. Claims data are often incomplete or incorrect. Examples abound of these problems as illustrated by physicians being downgraded for not performing a Pap smear on a woman who had a hysterectomy or a mammogram on a woman who has had a bilateral mastectomy. Litigation to correct errors like these is either threatened or underway in some places.[53-56]

Beyond serious process problems, however, are even more important questions about the concept of P4P. Insurers collate large amounts of billing information which profiles individual physicians by frequency and intensity of services provided. Physicians who see patients less frequently and have fewer intensive visits may receive incentive payments, quite aside from the needs of their patients. This process encourages some physicians to game the profiling system by avoiding the care of higher-risk patients. Physicians with sicker patients, especially those with impaired access and poor compliance, are likely to have lower profile scores even when their performance is excellent. This is because sicker patients require higher frequency and intensity of services.[57] Moreover, claims data cannot indicate whether or not complications of treated clinical problems have been averted by good care.

6. Information Technology

Recent years have seen many new efforts to apply advances in information technology (IT) to health care in the hopes of cost containment and increased efficiency. This trend is also seen as a means by which individuals and families can access Internet sources and thereby make more informed choices about their own health care. It therefore fits well with the philosophy of consumer-directed health care, and there is evidence that many people do turn to the Internet for health information. A 2007 Harris poll, for example, found that 52 percent of adults sometimes or frequently go to the Web for health information, as compared to 29 percent in 2001.[58] A new federal Office of the National Health Information Technology Coordinator (ONCHIT) was established in 2004 with a policy goal of reducing health care costs by up to 20 percent a year.[59]

Potentially very large and lucrative markets are attracting investors and vendors in the further development of electronic medical records (EMRs) and related Web-based resources. Examples include the very successful Web MD, Revolution Health (a new startup headed by Steven Case, AOL's founder), and Google Health (which is piloting an early protoype that includes a "health" profile for medications, conditions and allergies; a personalized "health guide" for recommended treatments, diet, exercise and drug interactions, and reminders for prescription refills).[60]

While there is no question that EMRs greatly improve communication and efficiency in many medical practices, especially in such integrated systems as Kaiser Permanente and Group Health of Puget Sound, there are many obstacles which will limit IT as a strategy for system reform. Only about 20 percent of patients have computerized records, which are mostly controlled by physicians, hospitals or insurers; detailed plans and performance measures have not been developed; there is limited trust between physicians, insurers, and digital record-keepers; and privacy concerns are formidable; already, more than 40 percent of federal contractors and state Medicaid agencies using EMRs have reported privacy breaches of personal health information.[61,62] Moreover, there is no evidence to date that IT can contain costs, and it may even turn out that it will lead to increased costs.[63-64]

Why Do All These Incremental "Reform" Attempts Inevitably Fail?

In a country as advanced as ours which claims commitment to equal opportunity and social justice, it may seem surprising that its chronic and entrenched problems (Table 6.1) are no closer to being managed today after many years of incremental changes. The last fundamental system reforms took place more than 40 years ago (Medicare and Medicaid). Since then, as chronic system problems fester and grow worse, one incremental reform effort after another passes from initial hope to failure. Figure 6.2 illustrates the inevitable results of these incremental reforms. How can we explain such policy failure? The following several interconnected reasons seem to me to go a long way in answering this question.

Figure 6.2
Incremental Change and U.S. Health Care

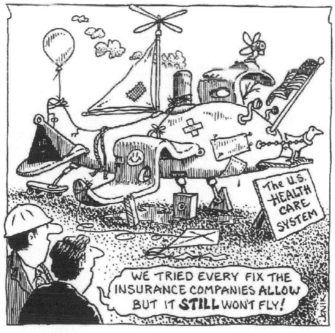

Source: Reprinted with permission of John Jonik

1. Disingenuous Disregard of History and Evidence

We have tried various market-based "reforms" time after time since the 1970s. Often they are promoted by their advocates as "new" thereby obscuring their past track record. Thus, we're now seeing a flurry of employer mandate initiatives by states at a time when that approach has been around for 30 years (Hawaii) without achieving universal coverage anywhere.[65] The politically popular CDHC and individual mandate "reforms" likewise lack historical credibility. As the current two major approaches to reform, there is little reason to expect that either or both can manage any of our major system problems (Table 6.1). Instead, we are almost certain to see increasingly unaffordable insurance premiums with less coverage, growing ranks of the uninsured and underinsured, further fragmentation of risk pools, erosion of safety net programs, and increased morbidity, preventable hospitalizations and deaths. Earlier chapters have documented consistently worse outcomes for patients as cost-sharing increases by insurers offering more restrictive coverage. Whatever cost savings are achieved by increased cost-sharing with patients ends up by limiting necessary care.[66]

2. Misdirected Targets for Reform

Another approach which assures policy failure occurs when reform initiatives are directed to the wrong target. Several examples make the point.

- Although intended to contain costs, CDHC and HDHI result in further cost increases due to patients delaying or avoiding preventive and necessary care, with higher costs of more advanced illness later on.[67]
- The unaffordability of health care is targeted by strategies that seek universal insurance coverage by private and public means, regardless of how inadequate that coverage is and without accounting for out-of-pocket costs.[68]
- High prescription drug costs are approached by privatizing Medicare, overpaying Medicare Advantage programs, and prohibiting the government from negotiating lower drug prices, even when the VA has already shown how effectively such negotiations can lower the costs of drugs[69]

- Under the guise of attempted cost containment of chronic disease, the drug industry is enabled to establish new markets through disease management programs that are largely disconnected from primary care.[70]

3. Ideologic Blinders

Especially over the last 30 years in this country, our approach to health care reform has been limited by ideologic blinders which assume that the "free market" is able to fix any of our problems through "market competition." We are told that markets will assure greater efficiency and value in health care as in other industries. This premise, however, fails to recognize the many reasons why health care markets are different from other markets, and that general theories of competition no longer apply.[71-73] The following are major reasons that dispell the notion that the marketplace can contain health care costs.

- 30 years of experience without cost containment
- Wide lattitude to set prices on supply side
- Perverse reimbursement incentives
- Deceptive marketing and advertising
- Consolidation among providers
- Oligopoly among insurers

The extent of ideologic blindness by market advocates is both enduring and appalling, as illustrated by these two examples 4 decades apart.

"Few trends could so thoroughly undermine the very foundations of our free society as the acceptance by corporate officials of a social responsibility other than to make as much money for their shareholders as possible."[74]

—Milton Friedman, PhD, 1967
Nobel laureate in Economics and author of
Capitalism and Freedom

(Concerning the continued uncontrolled inflation of health care costs)
> *"these are not signs that the health care market has failed. In fact – and it is crucial to understand this- they are the predictable results of vast distortions imposed on the market over decades. The government is the single greatest contributor to this problem..."*[75]

> —Representative Paul Ryan (R-WI), 2008
> Commenting on Report on Health Spending
> Projections through 2017

Another example of ideologic blindness involves the concept of moral hazard as a leading (if not the main) factor inflating health care costs. As we have seen earlier, this theory has been largely discredited as a principal cause of growing health care costs, and is now seen as much less important than other drivers of costs.[76-77] That the introduction of costly advancing technologies of little or unproven value into the market is a bigger cost inflator is illustrated by the explosion of imaging centers across the country promoting such screening procedures as total body CT scans, which also carry significant risks of radiation exposure while leading to further costs chasing down false positives.[78] Extending definitions of "disease" is another under-recognized inflator of health care costs. A current example is the lowered threshold recommended by the National Osteoporosis Foundation (NOF) and the American College of Obstetrics-Gynecology (ACOG) (both receiving support from the pharmaceutical industry) for screening and treatment of women over 50 years of age for osteoporosis. This will lead to new markets for drug therapy even without evidence that treatment will protect women from hip fracture.[79]

4. Hijacking of Attempted Reforms by Powerful Market Stakeholders

The Medicare legislation of 2003 (MMA) provides a classic example of the extent to which an attempted reform can be subverted by stakeholders in the medical-industrial complex. The problem requiring reform was the rapidly increasing costs of prescription drugs, much higher than in other industrialized countries around the world. Instead of dealing with that problem, the new law became a bonanza for industry, especially the drug and insurance industries. The MMA, dubbed the Medicare Middleman Multiplication Act by *New York Times* columnist

Paul Krugman,[80] was narrowly passed in the middle of the night after a full-court press by industry lobbyists and promotion by such industry-funded front groups as Citizens for Better Medicare (which opposed any price controls for drugs). A free wheeling revolving door between government and industry helped in its passage, as illustrated by the changing roles of Republican Congressman from Louisiana, Rep. Billy Tauzin. After chairing the U.S. House Committee which crafted the bill, a few months later he became President and CEO of PhRMA, the drug industry's powerful trade group even as he continued as a top lobbyist against price controls of drugs or importing drugs from other countries.[81]

The AARP contributed to non-transparent back-room negotiations with its own hidden conflict of interest. It played a key role in the bill's passage and had much to gain. Though little known at the time, about 60 percent of the AARPs income is derived from sales of its Medigap supplement insurance policies, sales of its membership list, and related activities.[82] A further conflict of interest was added when AARP sold its name as exclusive endorsement to United HealthCare Insurance Group, a major player in the new private Part D Medicare prescription drug benefit.[83] Meanwhile, of course, the private insurance industry was able to develop lucrative new markets through promotion of subsidized Medicare Advantage programs and HSAs.

5. Patchwork Approaches with Perverse Incentives

We have seen many examples in earlier chapters of perverse incentives throughout our health care system that lead to uncontrolled health care costs, profiteering through unnecessary services and administrative waste, and misallocation of services for our population. Each incremental reform attempt, as it seeks to address one or several problems on our problem list (Table 6.1), invariably runs into other unresolved problems which limit its usefulness. Figure 6.3 shows how intertwined and complex our health care system has become.[84]

Massachusetts again gives us a good current example of the need for more fundamental system reform. Even as the State works to implement its new hybrid employer/individual mandate law, those who become newly insured will have great difficulty finding a primary care physician. This is because reimbursement of physicians is so skewed toward some specialties that there is a serious maldistribution of doc-

Figure 6.3

U.S. Health Care: An Intertwined
Dysfunctional Non-System

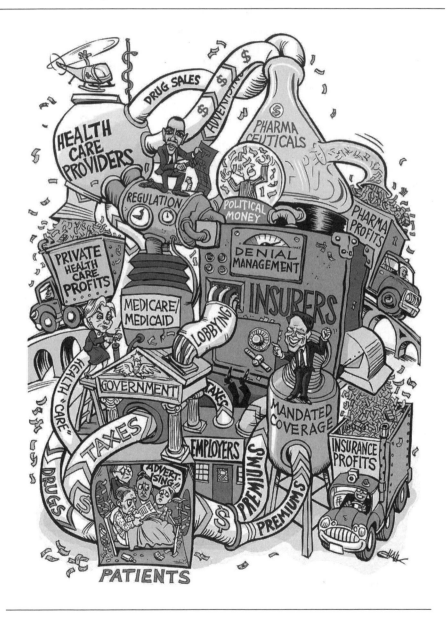

Source: Reprinted with permission of Tom Chalkley and *Tikkun Magazine*

tors. Only 51 percent of internists are accepting new patients, while 95 percent of the 270 general physicians on the staffs of Boston's top three teaching hospitals have closed their practices to new patients. [85] Nationally, largely as a result of distorted reimbursement policies favoring technical procedures and specialist care over primary care, declining numbers of graduating medical students are entering general internal medicine, general pediatrics and family medicine as our primary care infrastructure continues to unravel.[86]

Fundamental reform of physician reimbursement is long overdue and is essential if we are to rein in maldistribution of physicians by specialty. The income gap between primary care and other specialties continues to widen, driven largely by the more rapid growth in volume of diagnostic and imaging procedures compared to office visits. The median net incomes of most specialties are now at least double that of primary care physicians.[87] In his excellent recent book, *A Second Opinion: Rescuing America's Health Care*, Dr. Arnold Relman, former Editor of *The New England Journal of Medicine*, recommends that we abandon fee-for-service reimbursement and move toward salaried group practice in not-for-profit facilities.[88] This kind of change would likely make a powerful positive impact on most of the system problems listed in Table 6.1.

6. Retaining an Obsolete Private Financing System

Of all the reasons rendering incremental system reform unachievable, this is the most important. We reviewed in the last chapter the many trends which make the private health insurance industry unsustainable. Many adjectives describe its current state—unaffordable, inefficient, wasteful, deceptive, unstable, unreliable, and parasitic (as it skims off the healthier and more affluent and avoids the sick and poor). Private financing has become so complex in this country that another new industry is emerging—Web based companies that help patients to unsnarl and understand their medical bills. This adds yet another layer of overhead—and inefficiency.[89]

All of this is predictable. The costs, inefficiencies and inequities of private health insurance have been recognized abroad for many years.[90] A 2004 report from the Health Evidence Network of the World Health Organization concluded that: "Evidence shows that private sources of health care funding are often regressive and present financial barriers to access. They contribute little to efforts to contain costs and may actually encourage cost inflation."[90]

If the failing track record of the private health insurance industry is not compelling enough to make the change to a system of public financing, the growth of genomic medicine clinches the case. Robin Cook, physician/ writer and author of the 2005 book *Marker*, gives us this arresting observation:[92]

> *"In this dawning era of genomic medicine, the result may be that the concept of private health insurance, which is based on actuarially pooling risk within specified, fragmented groups, will become obsolete since risk cannot be pooled if it can be determined for individual policyholders. Genetically determined predilection for disease will become the modern equivalent of the 'pre-existing condition' that private insurers have stringently avoided."*

Where To From Here?

There are just two major options to reform the U.S. health care system—either continue to tweak our current multi-payer private-public financing system, with all its growing problems, or establish single-payer national health insurance (NHI) coupled with a private delivery system. We've tried the deregulated market-based incremental approach and it has failed for more than 30 years. Retaining a private financing system is incompatible with an affordable and sustainable health care system

With so many pseudo reforms bandied about by politicians and pundits alike, how would we ever recognize it if we were on the road to reform? Fortunately, we have some excellent principles and criteria as guideposts.

A broad cross-section of health groups, advocacy organizations, university departments and associations, unions, and faith-based organizations was convened in New York City in 2002. Their deliberations also included lessons from Canada, the United Kingdom, France, and Germany.[93] Their discussions resulted in these goals as a vision guiding fundamental system reform.[94]

1. Everyone should have access to the care they need when they need it, and without financial hardship (access, equality).

2. The cost of the entire system should not be excessive because everyone pays more when costs increase; costs should be controlled by eliminating waste, not by restricting effective services. Cost and access are related because when costs go up, access often goes down (cost, access).

3. Everyone should receive all the care that is effective in preventing illness and improving health, and no one should receive care that is ineffective or harmful (quality, equality).

4. Caregivers' work should be organized so that caregivers can serve the public to the best of their abilities under conditions that do not create undue job stress or burnout (caregiver friendliness, quality).

5. Health care should be delivered and paid for in an equitable way. People with more money should pay the same proportion of their wealth for health care (or a higher proportion) as people with less money, and everyone should be afforded equal access and quality (equality, access, quality).

Another set of useful principles was developed by the Committee on the Consequences of Uninsurance of the Institute of Medicine: [95]

1. Coverage should be universal
2. Coverage should be continuous
3. Coverage should be affordable for individuals and families
4. Strategy should be affordable and sustainable for society
5. Coverage should enhance health through high-quality care.

Although formulated by different groups at different times, these principles coalesce on such common ground as universal access, affordability, comprehensive coverage, continuity of care, quality of care, a population perspective, and public accountability.

Many studies over the years have already demonstrated that single-payer coverage can fulfill these principles. In terms of cost-containment and universal access, for example, different approaches to universal access, including employer mandates, individual mandates, and single-payer have been studied in many states. The results have been consistently favorable for single-payer as the only alternative achieving universal access with cost savings, while incremental approaches have failed to achieve universal access and cost much more in Massachusetts[96], Maryland[97], Vermont,[98] California[99], Georgia,[100] and most recently, Colorado.[101] Moreover, two earlier government studies have confirmed effective cost containment by single-payer coverage versus multi-payer market approaches.[102,103] Incremental market-based attempts to reform our system have consistently failed during the relatively good economic times since the early 1980s. We can be sure that they will fare even worse in times of economic downturn, and there are worrisome signs on the horizon. William Greider, well-known political and economic journalist and author of the new book, *The Soul of Capitalism: Opening Paths to a Moral Economy,* describes our current situation this way:[104]

> ..."the economy is profoundly unbalanced in old-fashioned ways: Wages and salaries have fallen steadily as a share of GDP, while corporate profits have hit a forty-year high. The Federal Reserve and its complicity with the carefree financial markets has pushed the rewards in one direction for roughly twenty-five years, and it shows. Financial wealth soared, while consumer incomes faltered and failed to sustain people's standard of living. As a national economy, we borrow to buy, both at home and abroad, and that elixir is losing its magic too."

A 2007 report by the General Accounting Office (GAO) projected "ever-larger deficits resulting in a federal debt burden that ultimately spirals out of control."[105] Meanwhile, the housing market slump and increasing defaults on sub-prime home loans are adversely impacting budgets of state and local governments[106] while many states are wondering if they will be able to pay for their retirees' health coverage.[107] By March, 2008, at least 25 states were anticipating budget shortfalls for the 2009 year, with California facing a $14.5 billion hole in its budget and Arizona confronting a $1.8 billion budget gap, 16 percent of its general fund.[108]

Robert Kuttner, founder and co-editor of *The American Pros-*

pect, co-founder of the Economic Policy Institute, and commentator on economics and politics over many years, describes our current economic vulnerabilities in these terms:

> *"A serious economic contraction could be triggered by any of several factors, which would then feed on each other—a softer dollar, higher inflation triggered by oil and food prices, a stock sell-off, a weakened housing market, rising interest rates, anxious credit markets, and tapped out consumers, most of whom have less real income and more debt today than in 2000. One cannot predict the precise sequence of events, or how steep the decline. But from the perspective of August 2007, it is painfully clear that all the elements of a severe downturn are in place, and that their common genesis is financial deregulation and speculation. The gross inequality of our era only compounds the risk, by removing one of the automatic stabilizers of that characterized the postwar era—broadly distributed mass purchasing power. And the unregulated global market makes it more difficult for nation-states to contain the damage.*"[109]

As we have seen in earlier chapters, the insurance industry and other corporate stakeholders in the medical-industrial complex have lobbied successfully for many years in support of market-based approaches to system problems. As the stakes and urgency for system re-design grow even higher, we turn to the next chapter to see how they are battling against fundamental reform this time.

References

1.   Truman H, as quoted by Stevens R.A. *History and Health Policy in the United States*. New Brunswick, NJ: Rutgers University Press, 2006, p 5.

2.   Sigerist H.E. A History of Medicine, Vol 1, Introduction. As cited in: Strauss M.B. (ed*)*. *Familar Medical Quotations*. Boston: Little, Brown & Company, 1968, p 215.

3.   Goldman D.P., et al. Pharmacy benefits and the use of drugs by the chronically ill. *JAMA* 291:2344-50, 2004.

4.   Davis K. *Half of Insured Adults with High-Deductible Health Plans*

Experience Medical Bill or Debt Problems. New York: Commonwealth Fund, January 27, 2005.

5.   Goldman D.P., Joyce G.F., & Zheng Y.   Prescription drug cost sharing: Associations with medication and medical utilization and spending and health. *JAMA* 298 (11):61-88, 2007.

6.   Artiga S. & O''Malley M.   Increasing premiums and cost sharing in Medicaid and SCHIP: Recent state experiences. Issue Paper. Kaiser Commission on Medicaid and the Uninsured. Kaiser Family Foundation, May 2005, p 2.

7.   Fisher E.S., Wennberg D.E., Stukel T.A., et al. The implications of regional variations in Medicare spending. Part 2: Health outcomes and satisfaction with care. *Ann Intern Med* 138(4):288-98, 2003.

8.   Relman A.S. *Second Opinion: Rescuing America's Health Care*. Public Affairs, New York: 2007, pp 91-2.

9.   Woolhandler S., Campbell T., & Himmelstein D.U. Costs of health care administration in the United States and Canada. *N Engl J Med* 349:768, 2003.

10. Smith C., Cowan C., Heffler S., Catlin A., & the National Health Accounts Team. National spending in 2004: Recent slowdown led by prescription drug spending. *Health Aff (Millwood)* 25(1):186-96, 2006.

11. Towers Perrin Health Care Cost Survey Projects that Average Annual Per-Employee Cost for 2008 Will Exceed $9,300. Stamford, CT: September 24, 2007.

12. Report of the U.S. Census Bureau, August 28, 2007.

13. Kaiser Family Foundation. Snapshots: Health Care Costs, Insurance Premium Cost-sharing and Coverage Takeup, February 2007.

14. Kaiser Family Foundation/Health Research and Educational Trust, Employer Health Benefits 2007 Annual Survey. Available online at: http://www.kff. org/insurance/7672

15. National Federation of Independent Business (NFIB). Decline in Employer Sponsored Health Insurance Traced to New Small-Business Owners. December 4, 2007.

16. Pear R. Many retirees may lose benefits from employers. *New York Times*, December 28, 2007:A1.

17. Kuttner R. *Everything for Sale: The Virtues and Limits of Markets*. Chicago: University of Chicago Press, 1997, p 114.

18.   DePiero A., & Kilo C.M. Will payment innovations benefit your practice? *Hippocrates* 14(12), 32, 2000.

19. Himmelstein D.U. & Woolhandler S. I am not a health reform. Op-Ed. *New York Times*, December 25, 2007:A35.

20.   Thompson A., & DeGolia R. Survey of 2007 proposals and initiatives
        by States by Universal Health Care Action Network (UHCAN) and the
        Progressive States Network. Available at: www.progressivestates.org and
        www.uhcan.org.

21.   Himmelstein D.U., Woolhandler S. Massachusetts" approach to universal
        coverage: High hopes and faulty economic logic. *Int J Health Serv*
        37(2):251-7, 2007.

22.   Felland L.E., Draper D.A., Liebhaber A. Massachusetts health reform:
        Employers, lower-wage workers, and universal coverage. Issue Brief No.
        113, Center for Studying Health system Change. Washington, D.C., July
        2007.

23.   Woolhandler S. & Himmelstein D. U. Health reform failure. *Boston Globe*,
        September 17, 2007.

24.   Gabel J.r., Pickreign J.D., & Whitmore H.H. Behind the slow growth of
        employer-based consumer-driven health plans. Issue Brief No. 107. Center
        for Studying Health System Change, Washington, D.C., December 2006.

25.   Knight V.E. A healthy aid to retirement: Investors seize on tax advantages of
        HSAs. *Wall Street Journal*, January 5-6, 2008:B2.

26.   Cochrane T. HSA funding. Are health care consumers leaving money on the
        table? Vimo Research Group Report, January 4, 2007.

27.   Stoll K. & Denker P. *What's Wrong with Tax-Free Savings Accounts for
        Health Care?* Issue Brief. Families USA, Washington, D.C, November
        2003.

28.   Relman A.R. The health of nations. *New Republic*, March 7, 2005.

29.   Berk M., & Monheit A. The concentration of health care expenditures,
        revisited. *Health Aff (Millwood)* March/April 2001, 9-18.

30.   Becker C. One question: credit or debt? As health savings accounts gain in
        popularity, insurers and the financial services industry want to bank the cash.
        Mod Healthcare 36:6-16, 2006.

31.   Woolhandler S. & Himmelstein D.U. Consumer directed health care: Except
        for the healthy and wealthy it's unwise. *J Gen Intern Med* 22(6):881, 2007.

32.   Ibid #18.

33.   Blumberg L.J., Holahan J., Hadley J., & Nordahl K. Setting a standard of
        affordability for health insurance coverage. *Health Affairs Web Exclusive*
        June 4, 2007.

34.   Dembner A. Older residents feel insurance law pinch: Age-based prices too
        high for some. *The Boston Globe*, August 17, 2007.

35.   Ibid #21.

36.   McCanne D. Comment regarding reference #17 in "Quote of the Day" July

26, 2007. Available at don@mccanne.org.

37.   RAND. Rand study finds health insurance subsidies won''t significantly cut
       number of uninsured. July 16, 2007.

38.   Gruber J. Tax policy for health insurance. National Bureau of Economic
       Research, December 2004.

39.   American Diabetes Association. High-risk pools. Health Insurance Resource
       Manual. Alexandria, VA, 2006.

40.   Girion L. Healthy? Insurers don't buy it. Minor ailments can thwart
       applicants for individual policies. *Los Angeles Times*, December 31, 2006.

41.   Families USA. AHPs: Bad medicine for small employers. Washington,
       D.C.: December 2005.

42.   Terhune C. Report raps association insurance. *The Wall Street Journal*,
       March 11, 2004, D3.

43.   Baumgardner J. & Hagen S. *Increasing Small Firm Health Insurance
       Coveage Through Association Health Plans and Health Marts*. Washington,
       D.C.: Congressional Budget Office, January 2000.

44.   Hoffman C., Rice D., & Sung H.Y. Persons with chronic conditions. Their
       prevalence and costs. *JAMA* 276(18):1473-79, 1996.

45.   Wagner E.H., Austin B.T., & Von Korff M. Organizing care for patients with
       chronic illness. *Milbank Q* 74(4):511-44, 1996.

46.   McCulloch D., Price M., Hindmarsh M. & Wagner E. Improvement in
       diabetes care using an integrated population-based approach in a primary care
       setting. *Dis Manag* 3(2):75-82, 2003.

47.   Fuhrmans V. Medco expands diabetes role. *Wall Street Journal*, August 29,
       2007:A9.

48.   Geyman J.P. Disease management: Panacea, another false hope, or
       something in between? *Ann Fam Med* 5(3):257-60, 2007.

49.   Holtz-Eakin P. CBO Director. Testimony to Congress. October 13, 2004.

50.   Mattke S., Seid M., & Ma S. Evidence for the effect of disease management:
       Is $1 billion a year a good investment? *Am J Manag Care* 13:670-76, 2007.

51.   Glickman S.W., Ou F.S., Delong E., Roe M.T., Lytle B.L., et al. Pay for
       performance, quality of care, and outcomes in acute myocardial infarction.
       JAMA 297:2373-80, 2007.

52.   Trude S., Au M. & Christianson J.B. Health plan pay-for-performance
       strategies. *Am J Manag Care* 12(9):537-42, 2006.

53.   Nakashima E. Doctors rated but can't get a second opinion; inaccurate data
       about physicians' performance can harm reputations. *The Washington Post*,
       July 25, 2007:A1.

54.   Rezzoni L.I. Assessing quality using administrative data. *Ann Intern Med*

127:666-74, 1997.

55.   Maclean J.R., Fick D.M., Hoffman W.K., King C.T., Lough E.R., & Wallter J.L. Comparison of 2 systems for clinical practice profiling in diabetic care: medical records versus claims and administrative data. *Am J Manag Care* 8:175-79, 2002.

56.   Stone T.T. & Sullivan D. "Tiering" physicians and "steering" patients. *Fam Pract Management* 14(10):24-6, 2007.

57.   McCanne D. Comment on Remes D. Exploring the nexus of quality and cost, August 31, 2006. In: "Quote of the Day," September 5, 2006 (Quote of the day /don@mccanne.org).

58.   Lohr S. Dr. Google and Dr. Microsoft: Two giants have plans to change health care. *New York Times*, August 14, 2007:C1.

59.   U.S. Department of Health and Human Services. Office of the National Coordinator for Health Information Technology. May 23, 2005, http://www.hhs.gov/healthit/valueHIT.html. (accessed April 27, 2006).

60.   Ibid #64.

61.   GAO (U.S. Government Accountability Office). Statement of David A. Powner. Testimony Before the Subcommittee on Federal Workforce and Agency Organization, Committee on Government Reform, House of Representatives Health Information Technology. HHS is Continuing Efforts to Define Its National Strategy, September 1, 2006.

62.   GAO. Report to Congressional Committee on Domestic and Offshore Outsourcing of Personal Information in Medicare, Medicaid, and TRICARE, September 2006.

63.   Wang S. J., Middleton B., Prosser L.A., Bardon C.G., Sparr C.D., et al. A cost-benefit analysis of electronic medical records in primary care. *Am J Med* 114(5):397-403, 2003.

64.   Sidorov J. It ain"t necessarily so: The electronic health record and the unlikely prospect of reducing health care costs. *Health Aff (Millwood)* 25(4):1179-85, 2006.

65.   Ibid #16.

66.   Ibid #6, p 3.

67.   Davis K. *Will Consumer-Directed Health Care Improve System Performance?* Washington: The Commonwealth Fund, August 2004.

68.   Ibid #33.

69.   Geyman J.P. *Shredding the Social Contract: The Privatization of Medicare.* Monroe, ME: Common Courage Press, 2006, pp 131-7.

70.   Ibid #48.

71.   Evans R.G. Going for the gold: The redistributive agenda behind market-

based health care reform. *J Health Polit Policy Law* 22:427, 1997.

72.   Nichols L. M., et al. Are market forces strong enough to deliver efficient health care systems? Confidence is waning. *Health Aff (Millwood)* 23(2):8-21, 2004.

73.   Kronick R., Goodman D.C., Weinberg J. & Wagner E. The marketplace in health care reform. The demographic limitations of managed competition. N *Engl J Med* 328:148, 1993.

74.   Friedman M. *Capitalism and Freedom*. Chicago: University of Chicago Press, 1967.

75.   Ryan P. Comment on Health Affairs blog February 26, 2008 concerning report by Keehan S., Sisko A, et al. (Centers for Medicare and Medicaid Services, Office of the Actuary, National Health Statistics Group) Health Spending Projections Through 2017: The Baby-Boom Generation is Coming to Medicare. *Health Aff (Millwood)* February 26, 2008.

76.   Nyman J.A. Is "moral hazard" inefficient? The policy implications of a new theory. *Health Aff (Millwood)* 23(5):194-99, 2004.

77.   Newhouse J. P. Consumer-directed health plans and the RAND health insurance experiment. *Health Aff (Millwood)* 23(6):107-23, 2004.

78.   Brenner D. J. & Elliston C.D. Estimated radiation risks potentially associated with full-body CT screening. *Radiology* 232(3):735-8, 2004.

79.   Herndon M.B., Schwartz L.M., Woloshin S., & Welch G. Implications of expanding disease definitions: The case of osteoporosis. *Health Aff* 26(6):1702-11, 2007.

80.   Krugman P. First, do less harm. *New York Times*, Op Ed., January 5, 2007.

81.   Lueck S. Tauzin is named top lobbyist for pharmaceuticals industry. *Wall Street Journal*, December 16, 2004:A4.

82.   Drinkard J. AARP accused of conflict of interest. *USA Today*, November 21, 2003, p 11A.

83.   Klein E. Drug beneficiary. *The American Prospect* 16(12), December 2005, p 8.

84.   Geyman J.P. Missing the boat on health care? *Tikkun* Jan-Feb 2008, p 49.

85.   Seward Z. M. Doctor shortage hurts a coverage-for-all plan. *Wall Street Journal*, July 25, 2007:B1.

86.   Tu H.T., & O"Malley A.S. Exodus of male physicians from primary care drives shift to specialty practice. Tracking Report No. 17, Washington, D.C. Center for Studying Health system Change. June 2007.

87.   Bodenheimer T., Berenson R.A., & Rudolf P. The primary care —specialty income gap: Why it matters. *Ann Intern Med* 146:301-6, 2007.

88.   Relman A.S. *A Second Opinion: Rescuing America's Health Care*. New

York. Public Affairs, 2007, p 156.

89.   Lawton C. New services help unsnarl medical bills. *Wall Street Journal,*
      September 4, 2007:D1.

90.   OECD (Organisation for Economic Cooperation and Development) Policy
      Brief. Private Health Insurance in OECD Countries, September 2004.

91.   Thomson S. & Mossialos E. What are the equity, efficiency, cost
      containment and choice implications of private health-care funding in
      western Europe? World Health Organization, Health Evidence Network, July
      2004.

92.   Cook R. Decoding health insurance. *New York Times,* May 22, 2005.

93.   Birn A.E. & Fein O. Why "rekindling reform?" *Am J Public Health* 93:15,
      2003.

94.   Bodenheimer T. The movement for universal health insurance: Finding
      common ground. *Am J Public Health* 93:112, 2003.

95.   Committee on the Consequences of Uninsurance. Institute of Medicine.
      Insuring America's Health: Principles and Recommendations. National
      Academies Press, Washington, D.C., 150-51, 2004.

96.   Brand R, et al. Universal Comprehensive Coverage: *A Report to the
      Massachusetts Medical Society.* Waltham, Mass: Massachusetts Medical
      Society, 1998.

97.   Sheils J.F. & Haught R.A. *Analysis of the Costs and Impact of Universal
      Health Care Models for the State of Maryland: The Single-payer and Multi-
      payer Models.* Lewin Group, Fairfax, Va, 2000.

98.   Smith R.F. Universal health insurance makes business sense. *Rutland
      Herald,* November 2, 2001.

99.   Kahn J., et al. Single-payer proposal for California as analyzed by the Lewin
      Group, 2002. www.healthcareoptions.ca.gov

100. Miller A. "Single-payer" Georgia health plan pushed. *Atlanta Journal
      Constitution,* June 22, 2004.

101. The Lewin Group. Technical Assessment of Health Care Reform Proposals
      (Proof Report) Prepared for: The Colorado Blue Ribbon Commission for
      Health Care Reform, August 20, 2007.

102. Congressional Budget Office. Single-payer and All-payer Health Insurance
      Systems Using Medicare's Payment Rates. Washington, D.C., April 1993.

103   U.S. Government Accounting Office. *Canadian Health Insurance: Lessons
      for the United States.* Document GAO/HRD-91-90. Washington, D.C.,
      1991.

104. Greider W. Waiting for "The Big One." *The Nation* 285(7):6, 2007

105. GAO. The Nation's Long-term fiscal outlook. The bottom line: federal

fiscal policy remains unsustainable. Washington, D.C., U.S. Government Accounting Office, GAO-07-983R, April 2007 update.

106. Merrick A. Housing slump strains budgets of states, cities. *Wall Street Journal*, September 5, 2007:A1.

107. Walsh M.W. A $58 billion shortfall for New Jersey's retiree health coverage. *New York Times*, July 25, 2007:A14.

108. Steinhauer, J, As economy falters, states facing budgets under stress. *New York Times*, March 17, 2008: A1

109. Kuttner R. *The Squandering of America*. New York: Alfred Knopf, 2007, p 105.

CHAPTER 7

Drawing the Battle Lines:
The Industry's Rear-Guard Action

"We are not real believers in the free-market mechanism unless we can honestly say that we would be willing to see some patients suffer the consequences if they could not afford an available treatment being provided to wealthier patients. If we cannot really accept that, then we simply will not let the market work when push comes to shove.

Proponents of the market approach also forget that an egalitarian distribution of health care is one of the factors that creates social solidarity, a feeling of community and the non-monetary attachments that bind a society together. If health care is not part of the social glue that holds us together, what is?

Health-care costs are being treated as if they were largely an economic problem, but they are not. To be solved, they will have to be treated as an ethical problem."

—Lester Thurow, PhD
Economist and former Dean of the
MIT Sloan School of Management, 1984[1]

"The United States subscribes to a business model that characterizes insurers as commercial entities. Like all businesses, their goal is to make money... Under the business model, casual inhumanity is built in and the common good ignored. Excluding the poor, the aged, the disabled, and the ill is sound policy since it maximizes profit. Under the social model, denying coverage to any member of society would refute the fundamental purpose of health insurance."

—Bernard Lown, MD
Developer of the cardiac defibrillator, Professor Emeritus at the Harvard School of Public Health, and co-recipient of the Nobel Peace Prize in 1985 on behalf of International Physicians for the Prevention of Nuclear War (IPPNW) which he co-founded[2]

Preceding chapters have documented what a mess our health care non-system has become. The public debate over options for health care reform has largely not happened. What little "debate" we've seen so far has been dominated by corporate stakeholders hoping to protect their interests in a deregulated market, their advocates, and theoretical economists. All of us, however, are patients somewhere along the line, and we are being adversely impacted by our growing health care crisis. The question now is whether we can mobilize the political will to deal with it.

As Dr. Thurow pointed out more than 20 years ago, our health care problems are not just economic but also ethical. Dr. Lown reminds us that the business model of health care builds in casual inhumanity as the common good is ignored. Together these two observations prompt these questions: what kind of a country are we, and what binds us together as a society?

In order to better understand the barriers to reform, this chapter has five goals, all aimed at analyzing what we are up against: (1) to examine the message being put forward by the private health insurance industry; (2) to outline some of the strategies used by the industry to delay or block fundamental reform; (3) to briefly describe the battle over the SCHIP program, as a case example of current political dynamics; (4) to describe how the industry allies itself with other stakeholders and coalitions to broaden its influence over policy; and (5) to briefly examine growing chinks in the armor of stakeholders' opposition to reform.

The Industry's Message:
Spin and Posturing of "Social Responsibility"

- *We believe now is the time for the country to meet this challenge head-on.*
- *We believe that every American should have access to health insurance.*
- *We believe that every child should be covered as soon as possible.*
- *We believe the health care safety net should be significantly strengthened. We believe employers should be incentivized to offer coverage to their employees.*

- *We believe those who have the means should be encouraged to obtain coverage.*
- *We believe that private coverage options should be exhausted before an individual turns to a public program.*
- *We believe access to health insurance should be a top priority for policymakers at the federal and state levels and that meaningful and sustained resources should be devoted to this priority in a fiscally responsible fashion.*

The above lofty language of beliefs attempts to convey the industry's commitment to its social responsibilities. But it isn't; it's slick PR spin from the industry's trade group, America's Health Insurance Plans (AHIP). The above *Vision for Reform*, released by AHIP's Board of Directors in November, 2006 goes on to say:[3]

- *We also believe that government alone cannot solve this problem. Health insurance plans, health care providers, employers, and individuals, all have essential roles to play.*

Taken as a whole this is a call to arms against any public solution to financing health care.

AHIP was formed in 2003 through the merger of the American Association of Health Plans (AAHP) and the Health Insurance Association of America (HIAA). Today, AHIP describes itself as the voice of America's health insurers, representing about 1,300 member companies providing coverage to more than 200 million Americans. AHIP's stated goal is "to provide a unified voice for the health care financing industry, to expand access to high quality, cost effective health care to all Americans, and to ensure Americans' financial security through robust insurance markets, product flexibility and innovation, and an abundance of consumer choice."[4]

The AHIP proposal for health care reform calls for expansion of insurance coverage for all children within three years and 95 percent of adults within 10 years through a private-public "partnership" costing the federal government about $300 billion over 10 years. Key elements of this proposal include the following:[5]

- Expanding the State Children's Health Insurance Program (SCHIP) to make eligible all uninsured children from families with incomes under 200 percent of the Federal Poverty Level (FPL)

- Improving and expanding Medicaid to make eligible all un-insured adults, including single adults, with incomes under 100 percent of the Federal Poverty Level.

- Establishing a Universal Health Account (UHA) to allow all individuals to purchase any type of health care coverage and pay for qualified medical expenses with pre-tax dol-lars, with federal matching grants for contributions made by working families to the UHA.

- Establishing a health tax credit of up to $500 for low-income families who secure health insurance for their children.

- Establishing a new $50-billion Federal Performance Grant to assist states in expanding access to coverage.

AHIP also promotes other means to work toward universal coverage, including high-risk purchasing pools, bridge loans for unemployed workers who lose their coverage, and tax incentives to promote broader coverage.

On the defensive over the kinds of business practices described earlier in this book, AHIP released a new proposal in December of 2007 as a further way to achieve universal coverage. Anticipating that more states may enact individual mandate legislation, the industry wants a greater say in how future mandates may be implemented. Its latest proposal recommends that Guarantee Access plans be established, whereby private health plans would be required to issue policies up to a pre-determined level of participation. But AHIP would like to set the bar for guaranteed issue at a very low level of only one-half of one percent of the health plan's insured population in the individual market. Premiums for such policies would be limited to one and one-half times standard rates. Karen Ignagni, AHIP's CEO, states that this initiative is "fundamental repositioning motivated by the Board's commitment to ensure that no American falls between the cracks of public and private programs."[6-8]

All of these approaches endorsed by the private insurance industry, of course, would perpetuate a deregulated private insurance market in its own self-interest while calling upon government to more generously subsidize private coverage. AHIP's recipe for "reform" relies on inefective incremental measures, such as tax credits, HSAs, and high-risk pools, which have already failed to advance universal coverage. The Guarantee Access proposal merely shifts more sick people to public coverage at taxpayers' expense. For all of the reasons we discussed in the last chapter, AHIP's recommended approaches lack any credibility as means to achieve universal coverage and also fail to recognize that affordability of the *total* costs of health care that confront individuals and families are far more important than the costs of premiums for insurance coverage of less and less value.

Industry Strategies to
Delay or Block Reform

Polls have consistently shown that by strong majorities Americans have wanted a single-payer insurance system for decades. In a democracy, how does the industry do such a stellar job of keeping this option off the table? As we will now see, the industry has many strategies up its sleeve as it defends its turf and future markets.

1. Lobbying and Campaign Contributions

As a non-partisan, non-profit rescarch group based in Washington, D.C., The Center for Responsive Politics has monitored lobbying and campaign contributions to elected officials and candidates since 1998. This is indeed big business. Total lobbying spending grew from $1.44 billion in 1998 to $2.59 billion in 2006. Over that period, the finance, insurance, and real estate industries led the pack. The insurance industry spent more than $130 million in 2006 to lobby Congress and federal agencies.[9] Meanwhile, political campaign contributions from health care industries to the 18 announced Republican and Democratic Presidential candidates have exceeded $12 million since 1989, with almost one-third of that total donated in the first quarter of 2007 and almost one-half of that to two candidates, Senator Hillary Clinton and former Massachusetts Governor Mitt Romney.[10] These increases in political spending coincided with the insurance industry's profits more than doubling from 2002 to 2006 from $20.8 billion to $57.5 billion.[11]

The effectiveness of industry lobbying is greatly facilitated by a revolving door between industry, government and Washington's K Street, the federal lobbying hub. AHIP's CEO, Karen Ignagni, is also a top lobbyist, as is Billy Tauzin, President and CEO of PhRMA, former Republican Congressman from Louisiana who chaired the U.S. House Committee that drew up the Medicare legislation of 2003 (MMA).[12] Figure 7.1 shows how frequently former members of Congress become lobbyists, in both parties, with top lobbyists receiving employment packages up to $2 million a year.[13-14]

The Council for Affordable Health Insurance (CAHI), little known outside of the insurance industry itself, gives us one example

Figure 7.1

Percentage of Departing Members of Congress Who Became Federal Lobbyists, 1998-2004 (By Year of Departure)

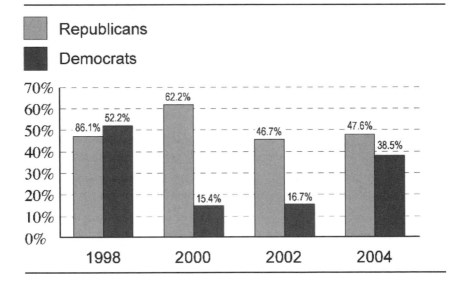

CONGRESSIONAL REVOLVING DOOR, ILLUSTRATED. Since 2000, with the White House and both houses of Congress in Republican hands, departing Republican members of Congress have had an advantage over Democrats in seeking well-paid lobbying work.

SOURCE: Reprinted with permission from: Guldin B. How to earn millions after Congress: Become a lobbyist and cash in. Public *Citizen News*July/August 2005, p 7.

of how the insurance lobby operates under the radar screen of public awareness. Since 1992, Washington, D.C.-based CAHI has been " an active advocate for market-oriented solutions to the problems in America's health care system as a research and advocacy association of insurance carriers active in the individual, small group, HSA and senior markets."[15] This group lobbied, for example, for expanded federal funding to support state high-risk pools, a major element in its ongoing effort to avoid state policies which force insurers to guarantee coverage and limit their prerogatives to raise premiums. Its advocacy helped to enact the High-Risk Pool Funding Extension Act by Congress in 2006,[16] despite the many problems encountered by state high-risk pools (egs., exclusions, limited benefits, high costs, and extended waiting lists.)[17]

2. Disinformation

AHIP's statements about its goals and approaches to "reform" are disingenous at best. When examined even superficially, its rhetoric is totally disconnected from reality, as these examples illustrate.

- AHIP continues to assure us that it is working to make insurance more affordable even as it steps up cost-sharing with enrollees and raises premiums at three or four times the rates of cost-of-living and median family incomes.

- AHIP promises more choice of coverage while failing to acknowledge the many circumstances under which choice of private coverage is actually reduced, such as in changes of in-network providers and hospitals, lock-in rules restricting enrollees from making desired changes at their own option (Medicare Advantage), and withdrawal of plans from the local market. And of course, the choice of what insurance plan you get and its cost can be completely out of the consumer's control, dictated by such factors as who the employer contracts with to provide the insurance, pre-existing conditions, age, whether the enrollee is a person or a family, and so forth. All these constraining factors disappear in a single-payer system, providing consumers with maximum choice and security, something AHIP neglects to mention.

- AHIP further claims that it offers more value in its "personalized" coverage while pursuing goals to keep its medi-

cal-loss ratios below 80 percent, if possible. A recent en-
trant to the individual market by Michigan-based American
Community Mutual Insurance belies such a claim—its new
two-tier "Coverage on Demand" plan targets the young and
healthy with a limited benefit plan that excludes maternity
care, anti-depressants and other services, has high cost-
sharing requirements, has an annual benefit cap of $5,000
unless "activated" by annual payments of about $10,000 a
year for a $5 million benefit cap that is subject to termina-
tion each year. It's easy to see why the company likes it; the
program projects an extraordinarily low medical loss ratio
sure to keep investors happy— just 70 percent (30 percent
of premium revenue for overhead and profits).[18]

- Without any new data, AHIP's Center for Policy and Research has attempted to discredit the methods and conclu-
sions of a landmark study, conducted by researchers from
Harvard University's Medical and Law Schools, of bankruptcies caused by medical bills. The Harvard study found
that about one-half of bankruptcies in 2005 involved many
middle-class Americans forced into bankruptcy by medical expenses, even though 75 percent were employed and
insured before their illness or injury.[19] The AHIP critique
argued, for example, that medical debts did not cause one-
half of bankruptcies and that the lack of adequate health
insurance could not be blamed as a major cause of these
bankruptcies.[20]

- Responding to a 2007 article in *Modern Healthcare* reporting that many attendees at a meeting of the Health Industry Group Purchasing Association believe that single-payer
NHI is inevitable within the next few years,[21] Janet Trautwein, CEO of the National Association of Health Underwriters, provides a mischaracterization of single-payer that
is both typical of industry public relations and is full of misleading assertions:

   *"Under a single-payer system, the government would
hold a monopoly over coverage, offering a one-size-fits-all insurance plan. So when the government decides to reduce or*

deny funding for treatments determined to be too costly, an individual has to forgo potential life-saving treatments, or finance them out-of-pocket. This is on top of the perilous problems other countries have encountered with this system, including substandard care, long waiting lists, loss of physicians, forced outsourcing and healthcare rationing. We need to consider alternative healthcare reform solutions, such as free-market reform, and just say no to single-payer."[22]

3. Deceptive advertising and promotion

One has only to recall the memorable "Harry and Louise" national television advertising campaign of 1993–1994 used to defeat the Clinton proposal, to realize the powerful impact of simplified mass communications. HIAA, then representing the interests of smaller insurers concerned about losing business to the five largest insurers, spent $14 million on that campaign, which featured a kitchen table debate of the Clinton Health Plan (CHP). The CHP was fatally flawed by its complexity, was a sell-out to the insurance industry, and would have failed to contain costs or achieve universal coverage. It is fortunate that it did not pass. But the "Harry and Louise" campaign, reflecting an internal battle within the industry itself, is widely credited with killing the plan.[23]

Today, as legislators in Congress seriously consider reining in overpayments to private Medicare Advantage (MA) plans, we are seeing another mass television advertising campaign launched by AHIP, which conveys the fear that 3 million seniors may lose their benefits if Medicare Advantage overpayments are cut. This disingenuous implication shifts the onus of responsibility to dispassionate budget-slashing bureaucrats, thereby changing the subject from MA's many problems. As we have seen in earlier chapters, these include deceptive and fraudulent advertising,[24,25] being more expensive and less efficient than traditional Medicare,[26] lack of assurance of claimed value of additional benefits,[27] and inadequate federal oversight of their actual performance.[28] Even the name "Medicare Advantage" is deceptive, implying superior benefits compared to traditional Medicare benefits, which if and when available require large overpayments from the government and would disappear if the playing field was leveled.

Blue Cross of California, owned by Wellpoint, the country's largest health insurer, is being investigated by state regulators for diverting benefit funds to excess dividend payments and rapid increases in its premiums.[29] It launched a \$2 million advertising campaign in 2007 against reforms being proposed by Governor Arnold Schwarzenegger and Democratic legislators, which include individual mandate and requiring insurers to offer insurance regardless of enrollees' health status. Through its political action committee with a misleading name, the Coalition for Responsible Healthcare Reform (Blue Cross of California is its only member!), it warns of unintended consequences of premium increases if such reforms are enacted, which could be comparable to California's energy crisis that followed energy deregulation. This approach drew the ire of the California Medical Association, which accused the insurer of continued profiteering without concern for the public interest.[30-31]

4. Courting of government even while disparaging it

It is an ongoing paradox that stakeholders in the medical-industrial complex court favors and markets from government while at the same time disparaging its size and role. The private health insurance industry thereby lobbies against restrictive regulation at all levels of government while milking opportunities to enlarge their share of public programs. In Chapter 5 we saw some of the ways in which the industry limits or gets around government regulation, as well as its vigorous efforts to expand its markets in SCHIP and privatized Medicare and Medicaid programs. In the aftermath of the release of Michael Moore's documentary *Sicko*, which called for elimination of the private health insurance industry because of its many excesses and lack of value, Karen Ignagni's main comment, as AHIP CEO, was an impressive PR spin: "discussion of the movie could advance the industry's interest in obtaining more government money for people who do not have insurance."[32]

The extent to which the federal government has accommodated the interests of industry, especially in recent years, is suggested by these two examples.

- The Medicare legislation of 2003 (MMA) created and funded the Citizen's Health Care Working Group, charged with the task of formulating recommended approaches to deal with problems of our health care system. After two years of community meetings across the country, almost one-half of the more than 800 participants supported single-payer NHI, by far the leading reform option put forward by the Working Group. Support for the free market as a way to ensure access to affordable health care ranged from none to 7.7 percent in the communities involved.[33] Despite its recommendations, however, the document submitted for further public review in 2006 ignored single-payer NHI and called for a system of insurance coverage of catastrophic illness with deductibles as high as $30,000, which was not even discussed in community meetings and was largely opposed in online polls.[34]

- Limits were placed on all federal agencies through an executive order signed by the President, published in the *Federal Register* in January, 2007, whereby political appointees are charged with supervising the development of rules and regulations by regulatory agencies. Defended by the Administration as a way to "provide guidance to regulated industries," the White House gained a gatekeeper in each agency to carry out presidential priorities and limit the authority of the agencies themselves.[35]

Meanwhile, of course, even as the private insurance industry seeks larger benefits and revenues from government, it takes every opportunity to disparage government with false accusations of "government-run" health care, alleged greater costs and bureaucracy, and less choice, efficiency, and quality than the private sector. Whenever the subject of NHI comes up, the insurance industry joins other stakeholders in the status quo with such scare tactics as labeling single-payer as "socialized medicine."[36]

The Battle Over SCHIP

The State Children's Health Insurance Program (SCHIP) was enacted in 1997 in an effort to expand insurance coverage for children in lower-income families. SCHIP built on Medicaid, has been funded through both state and federal funds, and allows states wide latitude in determining eligibility and benefits. By 2006 all states had created some version of SCHIP, with or without some linkage to Medicaid. Among these, 35 states set eligibility for coverage at 200 percent of federal poverty level (FPL) while 7 states set eligibility at 300 percent of FPL. SCHIP's original authorization was for 10 years, expiring on September 30, 2007. The debate over its reauthorization has become a heated battle involving state governments, Congress, President Bush, 2008 presidential candidates, special interests, and consumer advocacy groups. As John Iglehart, founding Editor of *Health Affairs*, recently observed: [37]

> *"Efforts by the 110th Congress, which is commanded by Democrats eager to reduce the record number of people without health insurance, coupled with other federal and state initiatives, have thrust health care reform into the political limelight for the first time in 12 years. Not since 1994, when the comprehensive proposal of the administration of President Bill Clinton was rejected, has the erosion of private insurance coverage and the continuing rise in health care expenditures aroused such intense interest among policymakers."*

The original 10-year federal SCHIP authorization was for $40 billion. In 2005, 11.2 million of children in the U.S. (8.3 percent) had no health insurance coverage, and states were finding it increasingly difficult to maintain their existing SCHIP caseloads. The 2008 federal budget called for an additional $4.8 billion for SCHIP over the next 5 years in addition to its annual funding of $5 billion.[38] A 2007 report by the federal Center on Budget and Policy Priorities, however, projected that funding level to provide less than one-half the funds needed by states to maintain their current SCHIP enrollments.[39]

The insurance industry and most conservative policymakers see expansion of SCHIP as a foot in the door for the dreaded publicly-financed NHI. As expected then, a battle royal has ensued over its reauthorization. The Bush Administration has offered an additional $5 billion for SCHIP over the next 5 years with the understanding that cutbacks of coverage by states may be necessary. The National Governors Association (28 Democrats and 22 Republicans) has called for expansion of coverage of the uninsured in many of their states. Democrats in Congress were quick to see the $65 billion in overpayments to private Medicare Advantage plans, together with a tax increase on tobacco, as good ways to fund expanded SCHIP coverage. The stakes of the debate over SCHIP thereby expanded to the future of Medicare, and an even bigger battle was joined pitting children against insurers.

In Congress, the House passed an SCHIP reauthorization bill by 225 to 204, which the non-partisan Congressional Budget Office (CBO) projects would provide insurance coverage for five million otherwise uninsured children.[40] The bill would authorize an additional $50 billion over 5 years for SCHIP expansion, in part by various provisions which would level the playing field between private Medicare Advantage (MA) plans and Original Medicare, including reductions in overpayments and a requirement that Medicare private plans spend at least 85 percent of their payments on medical benefits starting in 2010.[41] Following a protracted and intense lobbying and mass advertising effort by AHIP, including a threat that 3 million Medicare Advantage enrollees would lose coverage if the MA cuts were enacted, the Senate passed a bill (by a vote of 68 to 31) authorizing an additional $35 billion for SCHIP expansion, *without* the MA provisions.

Battle lines were drawn between the sides as President Bush promised a veto of any such large expansion of SCHIP. Supporters of SCHIP expansion include Democrats, the National Governors Association, the AMA, AARP, consumer advocates, and the public (a 2007 poll by Georgetown University found that 9 of 10 Americans, including 83 percent of self-identified Republicans, support expansion of SCHIP).[42] Opponents include embattled Republicans, the insurance industry (*unless* MA overpayments are retained), and the Administration. Although 80 senators reached bipartisan agreement to cover 5 million children through SCHIP, President Bush vetoed the SCHIP legislation, and Congress was unable to muster the votes to overturn the veto.[43]

After two Presidential vetoes of SCHIP legislation, the battle over SCHIP has carried over into the 2008 election campaigns, with Republican candidates raising the specter of "socialized medicine" and "class warfare" as the issue draws new inter-generational support involving advocates for seniors and children. The current Administration and Republicans continue to raise the specter of a foot in the door for "socialized medicine" if SCHIP is broadly expanded, and have worked to limit reauthorization funds and eligibility criteria to the poorest of families.[44,45] The irony of this position is pointed out by this observation by the Medicare Rights Center: "The same administration that wants to keep overpaying private Medicare plans (five-year price tag: $65 billion) has threatened to veto a Senate bill that spends roughly half that amount ($35 billion) to insure some of the nine million children who now lack health insurance."[46]

Allies and Coalitions
Against Fundamental Reform

As we have seen, the private health insurance industry is fighting a fierce battle to preserve and expand its interests in private and public markets. The industry is especially concerned about cutbacks in private Medicare plans and expansion of SCHIP as a potential forerunner of single-payer Medicare for All. In its fight against such a future, the industry naturally turns to other stakeholders in our market-based system as allies. These examples bring out both the diversity and common interests of stakeholders in the medical-industrial complex, though in a few instances these interests are at odds with those of the insurance industry.

Business and Corporate Interests
The large national public awareness campaign, *Cover the Uninsured* week during the Spring of 2003 involved town hall and discussion forums all over the country, and was supported by business and corporate interests as well as private foundations. Although it focused on the plight of the uninsured, it postured at reform by considering only incremental market changes without consideration of single-payer social health insurance.[47]

Employers
The little-known ERISA Industry Committee (ERIC) is a non-profit association "committed to the advancement of employee retirement, health, and compensation plans of America's major employers." It proposes continuation of private financing with a federal individual mandate and competing Benefit administrators in local and regional markets.[48]

Investor-Owned Hospitals

The Federation of American Hospitals, which represents investor-owned hospitals, has just released its own reform proposal *Health Coverage Passport*. This plan would expand coverage for Medicaid and SCHIP and add an individual mandate to purchase private plans, all with a view to give their hospitals relief from the burden to provide uncompensated care.[49]

Senior Citizens and AARP

With 38 million members, the AARP was a potent political force in enacting the Medicare legislation of 2003 (MMA), with its many provisions to privatize Medicare. Today the AARP is again flexing its muscles toward further expansion of private health insurance markets. Led by William Novelli, AARP CEO with a background in public relations who wrote the preface to Newt Gingrich's recent book *Saving Lives and Saving Money*, the AARP is adding more of its "branded" products to the market. For years it has dominated the Medigap supplemental insurance market through its endorsement of United Health Care plans. Now it brings to market three new AARP-branded products—Aetna plans aimed at the 50-64 age group; Medicare Complete, its endorsed Medicare Advantage Plan through Secure Horizons, touted as the only MA provider in the 2008 marketplace with a two-year commitment by the insurer (although premiums and co-payments can change after the first year); and its Medicare Rx Preferred, its Medicare prescription drug plan.[50]

AARP's main break with the private insurance industry has been its recent call, for the first time, for elimination of Medicare Advantage overpayments which the Congressional Budget Office (CBO) projects would save $65 billion over 5 years and $160 billion over 10 years.[51] AARP's credibility as a consumer advocacy organization, however, is discredited by its multiple unacknowledged conflicts of interest, such as its dependence on the marketplace for much of its funding, which prevents it from considering the merits of any system of public financing (which most of its members already enjoy through traditional Medicare). In 2006, for example, AARP took in almost $430 million in revenue from its branded products compared to dues income of $240 million.[52]

The Drug Industry

PhRMA, as the trade organization for the drug industry, and the private insurance industry were the main impetus and are the principal benefactors of the 2003 Medicare drug bill (MMA). Today, the two industries remain close allies in mining the Medicare marketplace for prescription drugs and insurance products. A 2006 article by Barbara Dreyfuss described the shadowy activities of three senior non-profit front groups—the United Seniors Association, the Seniors Coalition and 60 Plus—and a Christian evangelical group, America 21, funded largely by the drug industry.[53] PhRMA has launched national TV advertising programs intended to convey its social concerns, claiming that competition is working in Medicare, and touting its Partnership for Prescription Assistance (PPA) as "on the road to help you." Meanwhile, PhRMA carries on an ongoing disinformation effort defending expensive U.S. drug prices as the only way to compensate for "free riders" elsewhere in the world who rely on American R & D for new drugs, a claim that has been effectively countered elsewhere.[54]

The Tobacco Industry

As SCHIP legislation moved forward in Congress in 2007, to be funded in part by a tax increase on tobacco, the tobacco industry launched an intense lobbying and advertising campaign to block SCHIP and defeat such tax increases in a number of states. Tobacco opposition to SCHIP is no mystery when financing is based on a tax on tobacco. The American Cancer Society estimates that a 61 cent cigarette tax increase to $1.00 per pack would prevent 900,000 deaths from tobacco-related causes. The tobacco industry, however, frames the issue as "unfair to adults who smoke and to retailers who sell tobacco." This campaign by Big Tobacco led to defeat of tobacco tax increases in California, Oregon and Missouri while bolstering opposition to SCHIP by Congressional Republicans.[55,56]

Think Tanks

Citations of conservative or center-right think tanks outnumber those of progressive or center-left think tanks by an almost three-fold margin, according to Fairness & Accuracy in Reporting, Inc. (FAIR's) 2006 annual survey of think tanks. The leading conservative think tanks include the Heritage Foundation, the American Enterprise Institute, the Cato Institute, and the Hoover Institution.[57] They uniformly promote market-based solutions to health care problems, and put out many biased reports and recommendations with little regard for supporting evidence, as illustrated by these examples:

- The Heritage Foundation conducted a $30 million media campaign between 1997 and 1999 to discredit Original Medicare as an "inferior program" and promote and lobby for market-based solutions to the "Medicare problem;"[58] more recently, the Heritage Foundation published a preliminary analysis of the effect of state regulations on health insurance, concluding that excessive regulation will make insurance less affordable and add to the ranks of the uninsured.[59]

- The Dallas and Washington, D.C- based National Center for Policy Analysis (NCPA) is a well-funded think tank that describes itself as "a public policy research organization with the goal to develop and promote private alternatives to government regulation and control, solving problems by relying on the strength of the competitive, entrepreneurial private sector." Its Web site proudly proclaims its wide outlets to disseminate its studies and recommendations, including hard news wire service, television, talk shows, opinion columns in major newspapers, guest editorials, and releases to members of Congress.[60] In 2002, the NCPA published a 135 page report countering 20 "myths" about single-payer health insurance, using distorted evidence and unproven claims.[61] These "myths" have been rebutted elsewhere under 8 categories: access, cost containment, quality, efficiency, single-payer as solution, control of drug prices, ability to compete abroad (the "business case"), and public support for a single-payer system.[62]

The Media

It has been well known for years that only a few large corporations control all American mass media, usually operating across many industries as subsidiaries of giant corporations. In television, the 100 largest corporations fund about 75 percent of commercial TV time and 50 percent of public TV time,[63] with more than one-quarter of program time being allocated to commercials and non-program content.[64] Moreover, a 2000 survey by the Pew Research Center for the People and the Press found that 61 percent of investigative reporters believe that corporate owners influence news decisions.[65] As Ralph Nader has observed: (the major media conglomerates) are after all, "businesses that rely on advertising revenue and the goodwill of the surrounding business community."[66] These examples illustrate how these corporate influences prevent open, objective public dialogue over health care problems, priorities, and reform alternatives:

- When Measure 23 was gaining momentum in 2002 as a single-payer ballot initiative in Oregon, a coalition of insurance companies launched a campaign against it, blanketing the media with negative ads and outspending supporters of the measure by 30 to 1. With biased and inaccurate reporting, *NBC Nightly News* picked up on the insurers' claims without asking hard questions, such as how the costs of single-payer coverage would compare with existing coverage. No disclosure of any conflict of interest was made, although NBC is owned by General Electric, which is heavily invested in the insurance and medical industries.[67]

- In the 2008 presidential campaign, media coverage of health care reform alternatives virtually ignored the single-payer proposal by Dennis Kucinich (D-Ohio). Likewise, legislation for single-payer insurance, House Bill 676 (The United States National Health Insurance Act) which enjoys the sponsorship of 89 Congress people was similarly ignored.

- With web sites springing up everywhere with the success of Democracy Now!, and with independent film makers elevating documentaries to unusual popular status, the media landscape is changing fast. Cracks in the mass media's monolithic grip on what Americans see and understand are beginning to run deep, eliciting emergency reactions from the mainstream media. When the 2007 release of Michael Moore's documentary film *Sicko* forced reaction from the media, its coverage was generally biased and repetitive of myths; as examples, *USA Today*, CNN, the *O'Reilly Factor* and the *Wall Street Journal* warned of "government-run and socialized medicine," while Fox's Beltway Boys cautioned us about "a slippery slope from single-payer to a socialist dictatorship."[68]

- As expected, the more conservative think tanks are hard-wired into the media, maintaining a steady drumbeat of pro-market rhetoric. This recent Op-Ed by Betsy McCaughey, former lieutenant governor of New York and an adjunct senior fellow at the Hudson Institute, is a typical example of a scare tactic against the government's role in health care:[69]

(The health care proposals of Senators Obama and Clinton both) *"call for limits in the profit margins of insurance companies. Attacking the most unpopular industry in America may sound politically attractive, but if profit margins are legally capped, investors will flee to other industries and private insurance could become a thing of the past. That would leave only a government-run health-care system... Do you believe the nation should take that risk?"*

Some New Coalitions

In response to industry fears, we are now seeing a bevy of new coalitions in defense of the marketplace, sometimes with interesting bedfellows. Here are some examples:

- AHIP has been building the Coalition for Medicare Choices since 1999; its network now includes 400,000 senior activists, which lobbies Congress to expand SCHIP through the Senate's bill, thereby avoiding cuts of Medicare Advantage overpayments.[70] AHIP launched an intense lobbying effort through the political consulting firm Dewey Square Group, targeting 50 members of Congress, which resulted in the NAACP and the League of United Latin American Citizens sending letters to Congress opposing MA cuts[71]
- AARP, which is tied to lucrative private markets through Medicare Advantage and Medigap plans, has joined with the Business Roundtable and the Service Employees In-

ternational Union (SEIU) to "ignite a national movement, *'Divided We Fail,'* and search for solutions to health care" which continue to build on the private health insurance industry[72]

- The most recent addition to the new coalitions defending the health care marketplace is the National Coalition on Benefits. It includes more than 50 of the country's largest corporations and most powerful lobbying organizations, including AT&T, Xerox, United Health Group, Aetna, the Business Roundtable, and the U.S. Chamber of Commerce. A vigorous campaign has been started to lobby Congress to maintain their protections under the Employee Retirement Income Security Act of 1974 (ERISA), whereby large companies that self-insure their employees' health insurance are exempt from any state regulation of their health plans. Andrew McKelburg, vice president of federal government relations for Verizon Communications, summarizes the coalition's perspective in these words: "This is the one part of the healthcare system that's working."[73]

How Formidable is the Opposition to Reform? Chinks in the Armor of Market Stakeholders

There are growing signs that the defenses being mounted by the insurance industry and its allies to sustain their unfettered markets are less formidable today than they once were. They are being strained to the limit as a broad public backlash gains strength against the results of corporate dominance in recent decades. The 2008 election cycle shows widespread anger against repeated scandals of fraud and corruption in leading corporations, increased outsourcing of American jobs through a vision of globalization friendlier to Wall Street than Main Street, and tax cuts for the rich given higher priority than investments in our infrastructure (egs., bridges and levees) and social programs for the common good.

Because of runaway costs with no end in sight, the urgency for meaningful health care reform has taken center ring on the political stage, even in the middle of a war. And despite their massive funding, corporate stakeholders, think tanks, and the mass media have failed to create a majority against single-payer NHI. National polls have consistently shown strong majority support for NHI for more than 60 years. In the 1940s, for example, 74 percent of the public supported a proposal for NHI.[74] This number has ranged from 50 to 66 percent for many national polls since, even when the wording in these polls has typically suggested that NHI would be "government-run" (implying that the delivery system would not be private) and "financed by taxpayers" (without acknowledging the cost savings to be achieved by reducing the enormous waste in our private financing system). A large national study by the Pew Research Center for the People and the Press in 2005 showed strong support across party lines for a government guarantee of universal health coverage, even if taxes increase; among Republicans, 59 percent of social conservatives and 63 percent of pro-government conservatives shared this view.[75]

On one side of the political spectrum, we find advocates of limited government—the smaller the better—with emphasis on individualism and attitudes of social Darwinism—"if you can't make it on your own, you are morally less deserving." On the other end of the spectrum, we find support for responsible government as a means to promote the common good and an attitude that "we are all in this together." But we are likely to see more common ground across this spectrum as our problems get worse. The following recent commentaries insightfully describe where we now find ourselves as a nation:

"The modern conservative movement has embraced social Darwinism with no less fervor than it has condemned Darwinism. Social Darwinism gives a moral justification for rejecting social insurance and supporting tax cuts for the rich."[76]

—Robert Reich, Former Secretary of Labor
in the Clinton Administration and author of
Reason: Why Liberals Will Win the Battle for America

"At no time since the Great Depression have the working poor and the working middle class had more in common in their economic vulnerability, or been more in need of cross-class government programs, such as reliable pensions, health insurance, protections against income loss, and new needs of the broadly defined working family, such as child care. To the

extent that a class war is going on, it is the top 1 percent versus the bottom 80 percent. "[77]

—Robert Kuttner, Co-Editor of the *American Prospect* and author *of Everything for Sale: The Virtues and Limits of Markets*

"You have to respect the conservatives for their success-ful strategy in gaining control of the national agenda. Their stated and open aim is to strip from government all its functions except those that reward their rich and privileged benefactors. They are quite candid about it, even acknowledging their mean spirit in accomplishing it. Their leading strategist in Wash-ington, Grover Norquist, has famously said he wants to shrink the government down to the size that it could be drowned in a bathtub. The White House pursues the same homicidal dream without saying so. Instead of shrinking down the government, they're filling the bathtub with so much debt that it floods the house, waterlogs the economy, and washes away services that for decades have lifted millions of Americans out of destitution and into the middle class. And what happens once the public's property has been flooded? Privatize it. Sell it at a discounted rate to the corporations. It is the most radical assault on the notion of one nation, indivisible, that has occurred in our life-time. "[78]

—Bill Moyers, Journalist, Public Commentator, and author of *A New Story for America*

Our society has become so lopsided that even those who have spent careers benefiting from America's particular brand of capital-ism are becoming alarmed. Lamenting the erosion of stewardship and fiduciary responsibilities by many American corporations, John Bogle, former founder and CEO of Vanguard mutual funds and author of *The Battle for the Soul of Capitalism* observes:

"The age of managers' capitalism has had dire conse-quences for our notion of some sort of fairness in American society, and is a major cause of the increase in gap between

America's rich and poor, between haves and have nots. In the mid-1990s, for example, the wealthiest one percent of Americans owned about 18 percent of the nation's financial wealth. By the close of the twentieth century, the share owned by the top one percent had soared to 40 percent, the highest share in the nation's history, with the possible exception of the estimated 45 percent share reached around the turn of the previous century, the age of the Robber Barons—John D. Rockefeller, E.H. Hariman, Jay Gould, et al. Such concentration, most citizens would agree is antithetical to the long-term stability of our society."[79]

As a result of these trends, many Americans have lost confidence in the capacity of government to responsibly engage and manage major problems. The government's response to Katrina (FEMA and "heckuva job" Brownie) lend credence to that belief. Public concern grows as to whether we can solve our bigger problems. A 2007 survey by the Pew Research Center for the People and the Press found that the proportion of Americans who agree with this statement—"As Americans, we can always find a way to solve our problems and get what we want"—has dropped from 74 percent in 2002 to 58 percent in 2007. Other findings of the 2007 survey show increasing support for a stronger role of government in addressing growing inequities in our society, as reflected by these additional findings:[80]

- 69 percent believe that "government should care for those who can't care for themselves," up from 57 percent in 1994
- 44 percent say they "don't have enough money to make ends meet," up from 35 percent in 2002
- 73 percent agree that "today it's really true that the rich just get richer while the poor get poorer," up from 65 percent in 2002
- Today, 50 percent of the public identifies with the Democratic party compared with 35 percent who align with the GOP

The intense partisanship and political gridlock that we have now were not always so. This nation has successfully dealt with big challenges in our history, including taming and settling a vast wilderness, winning World War II, and pioneering exploration of space.

Perhaps the biggest challenge today is to rejuvenate and strengthen the capacity of government to work responsibly in the public interest for the needs of our entire population, not just the more privileged few. We have to get this right and soon. The increasingly dire straits faced by lower and middle-income families in gaining access to even the most basic health care have developed in relatively good economic times.

There are now worrisome signs on the near horizon that a serious economic downturn may soon raise the stakes even higher—the falling value of the dollar, high foreign debt, recent job losses, and bursting of the housing bubble are harbingers of more challenging economic times ahead. Dean Baker, Co-director of the Center for Economic and Policy Research in Washington, D.C. has these concerns:[81]

> *"The basic story is a downward spiral as the housing sector interacts with the rest of the economy: lower house prices, more foreclosures, fewer jobs in housing and less consumption, a weaker economy and less demand for housing. Throw into the mix declining state and local tax revenues due to the loss of construction fees and property taxes, and you have a further source of bad economic news."*

Previous chapters document the need for a larger role for government in the financing, not the delivery of U.S. health care. Politicians and political strategists tend to argue for incremental approaches to problems over any more fundamental fix. This is true of the current battle over SCHIP and with the platforms of leading presidential candidates in both parties during the 2008 election campaign. But we saw in the last chapter that all incremental "reforms" of health care have failed for more than 30 years. The time for more fundamental reform is at hand. In the next and last chapter we will turn to the kinds of real reform that are needed. Towards that undertaking, these words by Mark Schmitt, senior fellow at the New America Foundation and former director of the Governance and Public Policy Program at the Open Society Institute, are right on target:[82]

(as the debates go forward in Congress over SCHIP) "Democrats argue that the expansion is a modest one, largely intended to keep pace with population growth and health-care inflation. Republicans call it 'socialized medicine.' But then, they call anything 'socialized medicine.'... So, one might ask, if you're going to have to fight over 'socialized medicine' anyway, why not join the fight for an ambitious universal health-care program with a large role for public programs?... But public policy is littered with incremental changes that never went beyond the first step and actually foreclosed the pressure for further changes... Democrats need to remember this lesson, which the Republicans long mastered: Sometimes, it can be just as easy to win a big fight as it can be to win a little one."

References

1.   Thurow L.C. Sounding Board: Learning to say "No." *N Engl J Med* 311(24):1571, 1984.

2.   Lown B. Physicians need to fight the business model of medicine. *Hippocrates* 12(5):25-28, 1998.

3.   AHIP. We believe every American should have access to affordable health care coverage. A Vision for Reform. November 2006.

4.   AHIP. About AHIP. Web site accessed September 16, 2007.

5.   AHIP. Press release. AHIP announces proposal to expand access to health insurance coverage to every American. Washington, D.C., November 13, 2006.

6.   America's Health Insurance Plans (AHIP). Guaranteeing Access to Coverage for all Americans, December 19, 2007.

7.   Ignagni K. AHIP Press release. December 19, 2007.

8.   Abelson R. Insurers seek bigger reach in coverage. *New York Times,* December 19, 2007:C1.

9.   Lobbying database. Lobbying overview. Washington, D.C. The Center for Responsive Politics. Web site accessed September 16, 2007.

10.   Institute for Health and Socio-Economic Policy. Market-based Health Care: Big Money, Politics, and the Unraveling of U.S. Civil Democracy, June 22, 2007. Data from IHSP calculations of Center for Responsive Politics/

OpenSecrets.org data.

11. Institute for Health and Socio-Economic Policy. Market-based Health Care: Big Money, Politics, and the Unraveling of U.S. Civil Democracy, June 22, 2007. Data from IHSP calculations of SEC data, publicly traded for-profit corporations only.

12. Guldin B. How to earn millions after Congress: Become a lobbyist and cash in. *Public Citizen News* July/August 2005, p 7.

13. Birnbaum J. The road to riches. *Washington Post* National Weekly Edition. June 27-July 10, 2005, 22 (36, 37): p 16.

14. Lueck S. Tauzin is named top lobbyist for pharmaceuticals industry. *Wall Street Journal,* December 16, 2004:A4.

15. CAHI. CAHI issues: High-risk pools. Washington, D.C. Council for Affordable Health Insurance, 2006.

16. Ibid #15.

17. American Diabetes Association. High-risk pools. Health Insurance Resource Manual. Alexandria, VA, 2006.

18. Terhune C. New insurance plan has novel pitch -get sick, buy more. *Wall Street Journal*, September 14, 2007:B1.

19. Himmelstein D.U., Warren E., Thorne D. & Woolhandler S. Illness and injury as contributors to bankruptcy. *Health Affairs Web Exclusive* W5-63, 2005.

20. Lemieux J. Commentary: A cautionary note on the number of health-related bankruptcies. *Health Affairs* Electronic letter. June 8, 2005.

21. Rhea S. Universal healthcare crosses the partisan divide. *Modern Healthcare*, October 31, 2007.

22. Trautwein J. Why single-payer is not inevitable. *Modern Healthcare*, November 2, 2007.

23. Gordon C. *The Clinton Health Care Plan: Dead on Arrival.* Westfield, NJ: Open Magazine Pamphlet Series, 1995.

24. Pear R. Insurer faces reprimand in Medicare marketing case. *New York Times*, May 15, 2007:A14.

25. Williamson E. & Lee C. Medicare hard-sell. Abusive tactics found in sales tactics. *Washington Post National Weekly Edition*, May 21-27, 2007, p 24.

26. General Accounting Office. *Medicare + Choice: Payments Exceed Costs of Fee-for-Service Benefits, Adding Billions to Spending.* GAO/HEHS-00-161 Washington, D.C.: Government Printing Office, 2000.

27. GAO. Medicare Advantage: Required Audits of Limited Value. U.S. Government Accountability Office, July 30, 2007.

28. Pollitz K., Tapay N., Hadley E., & Specht J. Early experience with "new federalism" in health insurance regulation. *Health Aff (Millwood)* 19(4):7-22, 2000.

29. Girion L. Wellpoint dividend is questioned. *Los Angeles Times*, May 26, 2007.

30. Kurtzman L. Blue Cross funding campaign against governor's health reform. *The Mercury News*, May 24, 2007.

31. California Medical Association. CMA calls Blue Cross a leader in profits, not patient care. *California Physician*, August 9, 2007.Guldin B.

32. Freudenheim M., & Klaussmann L. Michael Moore's new movie takes on health care. *New York Times*, May 22, 2007:C3.

33. The Health Report to the American People. Report of the Citizens' Health Care Working Group, Appendix B, July 2006, available at http://www.citizenshealthcare.gov/recommendations/appendix_b.pdf.

34. Listen up! *Asclepios*. Your Weekly Medicare Consumer Advocacy Update. 6(32):August 10, 2006, p 1.

35. Pear R. Bush signs order increasing sway at U.S. agencies. *New York Times*, January 30, 2007:A1.

36. Krugman P. Health care terror. Op-Ed. *New York Times*, July 9, 2007:A22.

37. Iglehart J. Health policy report. Insuring all children—The new political imperative. *N Engl J Med* 357(1):70-6, 2007.

38. Ibid #37.

39. Park E. & Broaddus M. SCHIP reauthorization: President's budget would provide less than half the funds that states need to maintain SCHIP enrollment. Washington, D.C.: Center on Budget and Policy Priorities, 2007.

40. Krugman P. Op-Ed. A test for Democrats. *New York Times*, August 3, 2007: A19.

41. Medicare Rights Center. Cost-effective health care. *Asclepios* 7(29), July 26, 2007.

42. Krugman P. Op-Ed. An immoral philosophy. *New York Times*, July 30, 2007:A19.

43. Medicare Rights Center. Politics of health care. *Asclepios* 7(46), November 29, 2007.

44. Pear R. Children's health plan focus of new struggle. *New York Times*, August 1, 2007:A14.

45. Pear R. Rules may limit health program aiding children. *New York Times*, August 21, 2007:A1.

46. Medicare Rights Center. Cost-effective health care. *Asclepios* 7(28):July 23,

2007.

47.   Court K. & Flanagan J. Insurance "insurance reform"? Consider the source.
       The Wall Street Journal, March 18, 2003.

48.   The ERISA Industry Committee. A New Benefit Platform for Life Security.
       May 2007.

49.   Federation of American Hospitals. FAH unveils "health coverage passport"
       to insure all Americans. February 22, 2007.

50.   AARP. News release. AARP Announces New Relationships that Will
       Change the Health Care Marketplace and Improve Health of Americans.
       Washington, D.C., April 17, 2007.

51.   AARP. News release. AARP Opposes Medicare Advantage Inflated
       Payments. Washington, D.C., April 6, 2007.

52.   Stark K. AARP is drug plan advocate, marketer. philly.com, December 20,
       2007.

53.   Dreyfuss B.T. Poison pill: How Abramoff's cronies sold the Medicare drug
       bill. *The Washington Monthly* 38(11):23-9, November 2006.

54.   Light D. W., & Lexchin J. Foreign free riders and the high price of U.S.
       medicines. *BMJ* 331:958-60, 2005.

55.   Wayne A. Tobacco industry faces formidable opponent: Support for SCHIP
       expansion. *CQ Today – Health*, November 14, 2007.

56.   Har J. Health plan gets burned after state's costliest race. *The Oregonian*,
       November 7, 2007.

57.   Dolney M. Think tank survey. Think tank sources fall, but left gains
       slightly. *EXTRA!* 20(2):24-5, March/April 2007.

58.   The Heritage Foundation Media Campaign. Washington, D.C.: Medicare
       Rights Center. http://www.medicarerights.org/maincontentheritage.html.
       Accessed December 1, 2003.

59.   New M. J. The Effect of State Regulations on Health Insurance Premiums: A
       Preliminary Analysis. Center for Data Analysis Report #05-07, October 27,
       2005.

60.   National Center for Policy Analysis. www.ncpa.org/abo/, accessed June 28,
       2004.

61.   Goodman J.C. & Herrick D. M. *Twenty Myths about Single-payer Health
       Insurance: International Evidence on the Effects of National Health
       Insurance in Countries around the World.* National Center for Policy
       Analysis, Dallas, 2002.

62.   Geyman J. P. Myths and memes about single-payer health insurance in the
       United States: A rebuttal to conservative claims. *Int J Health Serv* 35(1):63-

90, 2005.

63. Korten D.C. *When corporations rule the world.* San Francisco: Kumarian
     Press & Berritt-Koehler Publishers, 2001.

64. Mink E. What ad slump? *Time Inside Business*, November 4, 2002, pp.A17-
     18.

65. Pew Center for the People and the Press. Available at http://people-press.org,
     2000.

66. Nader R. *Crashing the party: Taking on the corporate government in an age
     of surrender.* New York: St. Martin's Griffin, 2002.

67. Hart P. & Naurecker J. NBC slams universal health care. *EXTRA!
     December 2002, p. 4.*

68. Kao C. Diagnosis: Michael Moore. Media paint filmmaker as healthcare
     system's main problem. EXTRA! Update August 2007, p. 1.

69. McCaughey B. Op-Ed Health questions for the candidates. *Wall Street
     Journal*, February 20, 2008:A15.

70. Birnbaum J. In the Loop: On K Street. Health insurance industry looks to
     senior lobbyists. *Washington Post,* September 18, 2007: A17.

71. Lueck S. Private remedy. Insurers fight to defend lucrative Medicare
     business. *Wall Street Journal,* April 30, 2007:A1.

72. Stern A. An economic train wreck. *AARP Bulletin* 48(10):32, November
     2007.

73. Young J. Big Business launches healthcare lobby group. *The Hill,*
     November 6, 2007.

74. Steinmo S. & Watts J. It's the institutions, stupid! Why comprehensive
     national health insurance always fails in America. *J Health Polit Policy Law*,
     20:329, 1995.

75. Beyond Red vs. Blue. Report of the Pew Research Center of the People and
     the Press, Washington, DC: May 10, 2005.

76. Reich R.E. The two Darwinisms. *The American Prospect* 16(12):56, 2005.

77. Kuttner R. Thinking about the government. *The American Prospect*
     17(10):3, 2006.

78. Moyers B. Our story. *The Progressive* May 68(5):34, 2004.

79. Bogle J.C. *The Battle for the Soul of Capitalism.* New Haven, CT. Yale
     University Press, 2005, p 7.

80. Pew Research Center for the People and the Press. Trends in Political Values
     and Core Attitudes: 1987—2007. Political Landscape More Favorable to
     Democrats. Washington, D.C. March 22, 2007.

81. Baker D. The housing bubble pops. *The Nation* 285(9):6, October 1, 2007.

82.   Schmitt M. Every fight tells a story. *The American Prospect* 18(9): 9, September 2007.

CHAPTER 8

Beyond Denial of an Obsolete Industry to a New Day

"The health insurance industry is full of surprises, but history and experience show that insurers will never surprise us with a good, affordable health care system for America. No cocktail of regulations, subsidies and tax credits will provide health security to the uninsured, underinsured and anxiously insured—virtually all Americans.

Unlike private insurance, Medicare works for older and disabled Americans because it pools risk and does not punish people financially because they need costly health care services. It works because it has predictable benefits and offers reliable coverage. And it works because coverage is automatic, unlike Medicaid and SCHIP, ensuring all eligible persons coverage and protecting them against the risk of losing coverage for failing to sign up or recertify."[1]

—Diane Archer, well-known attorney, consumer advocate,
and founder of the Medicare Rights Center,
a national not-for-profit consumer service organization

We have spent too much money and lost too many lives over too many years to delay health care reform any longer. The time for real change has arrived. We can no longer afford to prop up an obsolete private insurance industry which provides less value all the time at greater cost. We need universal coverage that means something for all Americans at affordable cost—now.

Our health care system is falling apart, in large part due to an irrational and dysfunctional financing system corrupted by the business model. The private insurance industry serves corporate interests and investors before patients and their families, and is no longer worthy of the public trust. The time has come to replace it with a more efficient, more equitable system of public financing, coupled with a private delivery system.

This chapter has four goals: (1) to put forward a new vision for health care reform; (2) to describe what NHI will look like, together with other necessary reform elements as facilitated by NHI; (3) to briefly discuss winners and losers with NHI; and (4) to consider the current political landscape which may soon make fundamental system reform achievable after so many failures in the past.

Toward a New Vision
For Health Care

To counter the deceptive and wrongheaded frames of health care put forward by market advocates and conservative policymakers, the urgent need for a system of universal coverage must be reframed based upon long-standing American values. Based upon facts and track records of the two opposing alternatives to finance health care—multi-payer versus single-payer—the health care debate can be readily reframed on the basis of traditional American values. Here is how I would reframe the debate over U.S. healthcare:

> *Restore the promise of opportunity and security by promoting better health of our people, communities and country through enlightened health policies of fiscal prudence and fairness to all.*

National health insurance is not a liberal or conservative issue; it's an American issue. It's about delivering health care in the most efficient way possible. It's about eliminating waste. It's about making sure Americans get a fair shake for their money and aren't exposed to risk by loopholes in the fine print. And it's about making America competitive again, to be able to compete toe to toe with countries that use more efficient health care systems to protect their citizens for far less money than we spend now. Single-payer health insurance that covers everyone at a reasonable price spells opportunity and fairness that liberals talk about. It spells the compassion conservatives talk about. And it wins hands down over our current system as Table 8.1 demonstrates.

Table 8.1

Alternative Financing Systems and American Values

TRADITIONAL VALUE	Single-Payer	Multi-Payer
Efficiency	↑	↓
Choice	↑	↓
Affordability	↑	↓
Actuarial value	↑	↓
Fiscal responsibility	↑	↓
Equitable	↑	↓
Accountable	↑	↓
Integrity	↑	↓
Sustainable	↑	↓

In the 2007 Rockridge Institute Report on *The Logic of the Health Care Debate*, George Lakoff and his colleagues analyze and compare three types of political thought—conservative, progressive, and neoliberal, noting how neoliberal thinking (as illustrated by the leading Democratic presidential candidates) can fall into a Surrender-in-Advance Trap by continuing to propose failed market-based policies because of political opposition to the economically and morally superior progressive approach—single-payer public financing. They describe progressive morality as based on the value of empathy and responsibility for oneself and others, and call for a moral responsibility of government to empower and protect its citizens. They further suggest these progressive requirements for a health care system:[2]

- Everyone should have access to comprehensive, quality health care (follows from empathy).
- No one should be denied care for the sake of private profit (follows from empathy and protection).
- You can choose your own doctor (follows from empathy).
- Promotion of health and well-being, focusing on preventive care (follows from individual responsibility).
- Costs should be progressive, that is, readily affordable to everyone, with higher costs borne by those better able to pay (follows from empathy).
- Access should be extremely easy, with no specific roadblocks (follows from responsibility).
- Administration should be simple and cheap (follows from empathy and responsibility).
- Interactions should be minimally bureaucratic and maximally human (follows from empathy and responsibility).
- Payments should be adequate for doctors, nurses, and other health care workers. Conditions of their employment should be reasonable (follows from empathy).
- When people are harmed by either the unsafe practices or negligence of health care providers, the redress should be left to the courts—with no arbitrary caps on compensatory payments (follows from protection).

Elements of Fundamental Health Care Reform

There are eight basic elements for health care reform, as listed in Table 8.2. The most important building block is to establish a publicly financed single-payer system as an enabling structure to facilitate the other seven.

TABLE 8.2

Basic Building Blocks
For Health Care Reform

1. Single-payer national health insurance (NHI)
2. Evidenced-based coverage process
3. Reimbursement reform
4. Strengthening of primary care
5. Quality improvement
6. Transition from for-profit to not-for-profit system
7. Rebuild the capacity of government
8. Malpractice liability reform

Single-Payer National Health Insurance (NHI)

So what would NHI look like, modelled on a reformed single-payer Medicare-for-All program? Enactment of national single-payer legislation as represented by House Bill 676, now again in the Congress, would provide comprehensive coverage for all Americans without cost-sharing or other barriers to necessary care. Such coverage would go a long way in decreasing inequities and disparities of our present system while increasing the quality and outcomes of care. The health of Americans would rise, and they would save money compared to what they are paying now. Through administrative simplification, the intrusive bureaucracy of 1,300 private insurers would be eliminated, making available cost savings of some $350 billion a year for universal access to comprehensive benefits, including mental health parity, long term care, dental services, and prescription drugs. Future containment of health care costs would be facilitated by NHI's ability to negotiate prices set and enforce overall spending limits.

In one fundamental financing change, it would eliminate the excess waste, costs, and bureaucracy of an unwieldy private multi-payer non-system, replacing it with a more efficient, simplified system of public financing. It would assure access to necessary health care for all Americans through a private delivery system. Table 8.3 summarizes the main features of single-payer NHI.

Table 8.3

Main Features of Single-Payer NHI

Access	Universal access to all necessary medical care without cost-sharing or other barriers to care; all Americans receive NHI card throughout the country and U.S. Territories
Choice	Full choice of physicians and other licensed providers, hospital or other facilities in a private delivery system
Benefits	All medically necessary care, including primary care, emergency care, hospital services, mental health services, prescriptions, eye care, dental care, rehabilitation services, nursing home and home care
Medical Decision-Making	Clinical decisions made by patients and their physicians, not by invisible clerks and others in today's private insurance bureaucracy
Cost Savings	About $350 billion a year ($2,300 per person), mainly due to administrative simplification, monopsony purchasing, and improved access with greater use of preventive services and earlier diagnosis of illness
How Financed	All federal health program funds, such as Medicare and Medicaid, channeled into NHI program; remaining needs from payroll tax on employers (about 7 percent) and income tax on individuals (about 2 percent, but progressive by income)
Private insurance	Eliminate private insurance duplicating NHI coverage; retraining programs for those losing jobs in such areas as marketing, eligibility determination, and billing
Administration	NHI program administered by public or quasi-public agency as a single insurance plan with federal, state and regional boards; all costs paid by these agencies without billings to patients; global operating budgets for hospitals, nursing homes, HMOs and other providers; separate allocation of capital funds; adjustable budgets based on demographics, legitimate delivery costs, inflation, and beneficial new technologies
Accountability	Transparent public accountability; elected representation on federal, state and regional boards for governance and priority-setting

Source: Himmelstein D.U. & Woolhandler S. National Health Insurance or incremental reform: Aim high, or at our feet? *Am J Public Health* 93(1): 31,2003.

As we have seen in earlier chapters, Original Medicare has long been rated by seniors much more highly than private insurance, as illustrated by Commonwealth Fund's 2001 Health Insurance Survey (Figure 4.3).[3] But Medicare is not a perfect program. It has been weakened in recent years by privatization in many areas, including private health plans, the prescription drug benefit, and industry-friendly lax oversight by CMS discussed in a previous chapter. The Medicare legislation of 2003 (MMA) prohibited the government from negotiating drug prices as the VA does so effectively, while continuing overpayment to private Medicare plans without adequate accountability of reliable coverage. Enactment of Medicare-for-All along the lines of House Bill 676 would go a long way to remedying many of our system problems, as shown by Table 8.4.[4]

A comprehensive package of necessary health care benefits for everyone is made possible through cost savings in several important ways. A rigorous system for evidence-based coverage decisions will cut down on unnecessary services and those without proven efficacy. Large cost savings from administrative simplification can be redirected to patient care. Transitioning from a for-profit system run by corporate market stakeholders to a not-for-profit system will eliminate much of the profiteering that goes on today. As a result, such essential services as mental health care (with parity) and dental care can be extended to our entire population.

NHI will reverse the long-time trend of slicing and dicing populations into ever-smaller risk pools. It will do the reverse of cherry picking. Instead of casting aside the ill and those most in need of health insurance, NHI will do what insurance is supposed to do— spread the risk across 300 million Americans, rather than concentrate it as private health insurance has done into the lucky few who are for a time both younger and healthier than many of us. The argument against this is that it will unfairly cost the healthy more because part of their tax dollars would go to taking care of the ill. But this is a false equation. Yes, money goes to take care of the sick, but it costs less to insure everyone this way than with our current system; costs will drop, not rise.

With the elimination of financial barriers to care, patients will have free choice of physicians and other licensed providers for all necessary care, including approved preventive and screening services. Administrative hassles will be largely resolved, no longer requiring

TABLE 8.4

A Problem-Oriented Approach to System Reform

PROBLEM	ACTION
1. Uncontrolled inflation of health care costs and prices	Advocate for single-payer National Health Insurance (NHI), Medicare for All, a publicly financed program of comprehensive health insurance coupled with a private delivery system; lower overhead and improved efficiency by risk pooling across our entire population. NHI would consolidate health care programs, simplify administration, and provide the structure for more accountability to the system.
2. Growing crisis in unaffordability of health care now extending to middle class	
3. Decreasing access to care	
4. Rising rates of uninsured and underinsured	
5. Gaps in coverage for essential services	
6. 29-month waiting period for coverage of disabled on Medicare	
7. Lack of mental health parity	
8. Discontinuity and turnover of insurance coverage	
9. Variable, often poor quality of care	
10. High rates of inappropriate and unnecessary care	
11. Increasing health disparities	
12. Administrative complexity, profiteering and waste of 1,300 private insurers	
13. Decreased choice of hospital and physician in managed care programs	
14. Erosion of safety net programs	
15. Lax federal regulation of drug, medical device, and dietary supplement industries	Advocate for expanded authority and resources for FDA and support its independence from political interference.
16. Inadequate national system for assessment of new medical technologies	Support creation of new federal agency for this purpose, possibly along the lines of the National Transportation Safety Board.
17. Declining primary care base	Support narrowing of reimbursement gap between procedural and cognitive health care services, together with other policies to expand training programs and strengthen the delivery model for primary care physicians.

Source: Geyman, J.P. *The Corrosion of Medicine: Can the Profession Reclaim its Moral Legacy?* Monroe, ME. Common Courage Press, 2008, p216

transactions with 1,300 private insurers and many thousands of different policies. With their annually-negotiated global budgets, hospitals can eliminate most of their costly billing departments, freeing up funds for patient care.

With annual health care expenditures exceeding $2.2 trillion in by far the most expensive system in the world, there is plenty of money in the system to provide universal coverage if re-channeled wisely. The government already spends 64 percent of the total, including federal health programs, tax exceptions, and disproportionate share payments to hospitals for uncompensated care. With all of these funds redirected to Medicare-for-All, the remainder is raised through a payroll tax on employers of 7.7 percent (less than their present 8.5 percent average currently paid to private insurance companies) and an income tax averaging 2 percent for most taxpayers. This 2 percent tax burden will be balanced by not having to pay larger costs under our present system, including insurance premiums, co-payments, deductibles, and other out-of-pocket payments. This kind of financing effectively rebuts conservative claims that a single-payer system will require us to pay more than we now pay for health care.

Single-payer NHI will bring to bear new ways to contain health care costs even while assuring universal coverage. First, of course, are the huge administrative savings; the overhead for Medicare (despite its current problems) now averages only about 3 percent compared to an average of 18 percent for commercial insurers and as much as 26.5 percent for investor-owned Blues.[5] Monopsony purchasing (bulk purchasing by a single-payer) of drugs, medical devices, and supplies provides a second way to conserve funds. Negotiated fees with physicians and other providers, together with negotiated global budgets with hospitals and other facilities, provides a third mechanism to wring waste and profiteering out of the system.

In today's multi-payer system, public policy is largely set by insurers and other corporate stakeholders, with little transparency or opportunities to redress problems. Single-payer NHI will provide more transparency and involvement of the public in policy making. Each state will have an elected and appointed body representing the people of the state. This body will be responsible for decisions on the benefit package and new technologies (working with advisory groups of health care professionals), health planning, priority setting, and negotiation of professional fees and facility budgets.

Other Necessary Elements of Health Care Reform

Although change from a multi-payer private-public system of financing to a publicly-financed single-payer system is by far the single most important requirement for lasting system reform, single-payer NHI by itself will not remedy all of our problems. These other elements of reform will also be required, each working interactively to make others more effective and each in turn made more achievable by single-payer financing.

1. Evidence-Based Coverage Process

While it would seem to be uncontroversial to base all coverage decisions on the best scientific evidence available, industry stakeholders have fought vigorously for many years against evidence-based criteria. The drug and medical device industries, for example, far prefer a rapid and industry-friendly approach by the FDA in the approval of new products. They have successfully lobbied for many years against the use of cost-effectiveness as a criterion in the approval process. As a result, a 1999 report by the Technology Evaluation Committee of Blue Cross Blue Shield found that nearly one-third of evaluations of drugs, medical devices, or procedures were lacking or uncertain in their effectiveness.[6] Many new drugs are not really better, just heavily marketed, more expensive "me too" drugs (egs., Nexium versus Prilosec, Clarinex versus Claritin). A 2003 report from the Health Research Group of Public Citizen evaluated seven pairs of drugs, finding that six had no therapeutic advantage over its predecessor, with one more toxic than the original.[7]

Industry opposition succeeded in dismantling earlier efforts by the federal government to establish a national body for technology assessment, such as the National Center for Technology Assessment (1978-1981). Conservative legislators responded to industry's concerns in the 1990s by neutering the Agency for Health Care Policy and Research (AHCPR), cutting back its roles and funding while excising "Policy" from its new name, the Agency for Healthcare Research and Quality (AHRQ).[8] In reaction to Medicare's issuance of a Notice of Intent (NOI) in 2000 that would require new technologies to demonstrate "medical benefit" as well as "added value," industry mobilized professional groups, consumer advocates, and other organizations in a successful campaign against the use of such criteria, especially the use of cost-effectiveness.[9] A strong multidisciplinary federal body of experts is long overdue to make national coverage decisions, independent of corporate and political influence, perhaps modelled along the lines of the U.S. Federal Reserve Board.[10]

2. Reimbursement Reform

Renegotiation of physician fee schedules is one of the first orders of business as NHI is implemented. This process offers two big opportunities to rein in health care costs: (1) by narrowing the wide gap between reimbursement of procedural and cognitive services provided by physicians; and (2) by elimination of unreasonable differences in reimbursement patterns which have developed over the last 40 years in the Medicare program from one part of the country to another. These two factors have contributed in large part to specialty and geographic maldistribution of physicians, despite the best efforts of the medical education community to address the problem.

As we have seen in earlier chapters, physicians are attracted to the best paid specialties and to higher-reimbursed parts of the country, with overuse of many inappropriate and unnecessary services due to physician-induced demand.[11] Many procedures are currently over-reimbursed while cognitive services typical in primary care (ie., the face-to-face listening and talking part of medicine, including coordination and continuity of comprehensive care), are under-reimbursed.

Reimbursement reform can help to limit maldistribution of physicians as well as inappropriate physician-induced demand. Medicine's generalist base is disappearing as an unintended consequence of our current reimbursement system based on the resource-based relative value scale (RBRVS)[12] that allows much higher reimbursement for procedures and specialist care than for preventive, diagnostic and management services by primary care physicians. Based on their comprehensive recent analysis of the primary care-specialty income gap, Drs. Bodenheimer, Berenson and Rudolf recommend that new payment models be developed that blend the best of fee-for-service, capitation and salary while mitigating the problems of each approach.[13]

3. Strengthening of Primary Care

A strong primary care base is essential to any health care system for access, provision and coordination of comprehensive health care. Countries with strong primary care have at least one-half of their physicians in primary care (egs., 50 percent in Canada, 70 percent in the United Kingdom),[14] enabling them to have lower overall health care costs, improved health outcomes and healthier populations. By comparison, fewer than 30 percent of American physicians today are in primary care specialties.

As the most general of all specialties, family physicians are also the most widely dispersed in urban, suburban, rural and underserved parts of the country.[15] Many studies have shown that generalist physicians provide more comprehensive and cost-effective care than physicians in non-primary care fields, typically with increased likelihood to recognize mental health disorders, more sparing use of technology, lower rates of hospitalization, and better quality of care.[16-20] The 2006 Health Care Quality Survey of the Commonwealth Fund concluded that a medical home in primary care can lead to higher rates of preventive screening and reduce or even eliminate racial and ethnic disparities in access and quality of care.[21]

The growing gap between procedure-based reimbursement of physician services and cognitive services more typical in primary care has led to an increasing national shortage of primary care and some other specialties, such as psychiatry. Physician maldistribution by specialty and geography has become a critical problem despite efforts within the medical education community to address the problem. The number of U.S. medical graduates choosing family medicine has declined by 50 percent over the last 10 years, only 20 percent internal medicine residents become general internists, and most pediatricians also favor subspecialties over generalist practice.[22] Meanwhile, medical graduates flock into such high-income specialties as radiology, orthopedic surgery, and anesthesiology with incomes two or three times higher than in the primary care specialties.[23]

Reimbursement for primary care services needs to be increased if family medicine, general internal medicine, and general pediatrics are to rejuvenate themselves and become capable of providing universal access to necessary care for our entire population in a reformed system. With NHI, primary care reimbursement is likely to increase while that of many non-primary care services will be reduced.

Specialists in non-primary care fields are ill prepared to provide primary care, either by training, expertise or commitment. While there is to some extent a "hidden system" whereby some specialists care for some problems outside their field, this is hardly a solid base upon which to build a health care system.[24]

The advent of NHI will further strain our already weakened primary care base, which has suffered as graduating medical students seek more attractive lifestyles in higher-income non-primary care fields. The American College of Physicians, the second largest medical organization in this country, has recently warned that our primary care infrastructure is "at grave risk of collapse,"[25] and has endorsed single-payer NHI as one of two major options to reform our system.[26]

It will take a serious, high priority multifaceted effort to rebuild primary care to meet the nation's needs. A 2006 report by the AMA's Council on Medical Education called for steps to foster the Medical Home in the primary care specialties and reimbursement changes to make generalist careers more attractive.[27] Other strategies to strengthen primary care could well include development of loan forgiveness programs for graduating medical students entering primary care residencies (average debt today at graduation exceeds $105,000 in public medical schools and $140,000 in private medical schools)[28]; increased funding of graduate medical education (GME) in primary care; and reallocation of GME training slots by specialty.

4. Quality Improvement

As we saw in Chapter 4, the U.S. compares poorly with many other industrialized countries around the world in terms of health outcomes and quality of care benchmarks, despite spending far more on health care than any other country.[29-31] Quality of care tends to be lower in areas with larger proportions of specialists, more use of medical technology, and larger amounts of unnecessary and inappropriate care.[32-34]

NHI can lead to improved quality of care in several important and inter-related ways, including (1) universal access to necessary care without financial barriers; (2) expanded use of preventive care, earlier diagnosis and treatment of disease, and chronic disease management integrated in primary care settings; (3) aligning economic incentives with best practice; (4) reimbursement policies informed by evidence-based technology assessment (including non-payment for such un-proven and potentially harmful services as total body CT scanning as a screening procedure); (5) expanded use of information management systems and electronic medical records in a simplified administrative system; and (6) monitoring and analysis of regional and national per-formance data of utilization and quality markers.

5. Transition from For-Profit to Not-For-Profit System

Moving from today's investor-owned for-profit system towards a not-for-profit system is required if we are to successfully rein in con-tinued inflation of health care costs and improve the quality of care. Enormous cost savings will be realized by replacing for-profit private insurers with a single public payer. In our corporate market-based sys-tem, financial self-interest that maximizes return to shareholders has become the norm throughout today's system, whether private insurers, the drug or medical device industries.[35] As Relman observes:[36]

"In my view, an insufficiently recognized cause of medi-cal inflation in the U.S. is the extent of the entrepreneurialism and commercialism in the medical care delivery system. That is what distinguishes the U.S. from all other advanced countries and that is what largely accounts for our having the highest rate of inflation in health costs. To control this economic drive to maximize income, we need to change the economic incen-tives for doctors, since they order almost all medical services. We will also have to discourage investor-ownership of health care, because it is a powerful stimulus for continued increase in the income of health care providers."

Beyond the cost problem, investor-owned care is also of lower quality, whether hospitals, HMOs, nursing homes, dialysis centers, or mental health facilities.[37]

NHI will provide a structure within which to transition away from health care as a commodity to an essential public good. Prices will be negotiated with manufacturers and suppliers based on their real costs, exclusive of their advertising, marketing, and lobbying costs. Regional health planning boards will allocate capital funds for the construction of facilities and purchase of expensive technologies based on regional needs. Investor-owned facilities and providers will be converted over a transitional period of 10 to 15 years to not-for-profit status. Long-term bonds will be issued by the NHI program in order to amortize the one-time costs of compensating investors for the appraisal value of their facilities.

Some of our best HMOs, such as Kaiser Permanente and Group Health Cooperative, are already not-for-profit and will serve as models for private health plan conversions. A major effort will be made to re-train displaced workers from the private insurance industry and place them in other health-related jobs.[38]

6. Rebuild the Capacity of Government

Our many years of profit-driven governance have weakened government by outsourcing many of its functions to private interests with lax oversight, underfunding of regulatory agencies, cronyism and revolving doors of leadership between government, K Street and in-dustry, and frank incompetence (eg., Brownie, FEMA, and Katrina). As Michael Lipsky and Dianne Stewart of Public Works, a Program of Dèmos, recently observed:[39]

> *"Public opinion toward government has been shaped by decades of relentless negative rhetoric, emphasizing gov-ernment waste and mismanagement. Political leaders of both parties contribute to this dysfunctional perspective, running against government when campaigning and then criticizing government rather than championing its necessary role once they're in office. This cynicism has brought the public to a point that it has trouble even imagining the creation of effective pub-lic structures to manage the people's business."*

We have had 20 years of Republican governance with a consis-tent goal to nurture private markets and downsize government. As an example of this conservative ideology, Paul O'Neill, as Secretary of the Treasury and previously a top executive at two large multinational corporations, suggested in 2001 that:

> *"...corporations should be tax-exempt, like churches, and that Social Security, Medicare, and Medicaid should be eliminated since able-bodied adults should save enough on a*

*regular basis so that they can provide for their own retirement,
and for that matter, health and medical needs.* "[40]

The philosophy of Grover Norquist, lobbyist and president of Americans for Tax Reform, is equally clear:

*"I don't want to abolish government. I simply want to
reduce it to the size where I can drag it into the bathroom and
drown it in the bathtub."*[41]

As part of its policy goal to privatize and downsize government over the last 7 years, the government itself contributes to the growing ranks of the uninsured. In the same way that many corporations outsource jobs overseas in order to pay lower wages and avoid the burden of paying for benefits, the federal government also plays that game. According to Paul Light, PhD, Professor of Public Service at New York University's Wagner Graduate School of Public Service, the U. S. government outsourced 5.4 million federal-contract workers in 2005, double the number in 1990. About 80 percent of these are lower-wage workers, who are least likely to be offered or to obtain health insurance. The government has no way of tracking how many have health insurance. A 2007 investigation by the Labor Department found that employers failed to pay proper wages or provide benefits or both in 80 percent of these cases.[42]

Ironical and cynical as it is, conservatives in government have been pushing to privatize and weaken Medicare since the Contract with America was first introduced in 1995 by the new Republican majority in Congress. The goal was to "save" the program by killing it. As Speaker of the House Newt Gingrich said at the time, this kind of "reform" could result in "solving the Medicare problem" by leading it to "wither on the vine."[43] The plan, of course, was to skim off healthier seniors to subsidized private plans leaving the traditional Medicare program with more costly sicker patients and increased risk to fall into a death spiral due to adverse selection. Princeton's Uwe Reinhardt concluded that the most likely goal of conservative legislators and politicians is to "reduce the payer's exposure to Medicare spending, even if it increased total health spending per Medicare beneficiary."[44]

It will not be easy to rid ourselves of undue influence over public policy by vested interests. Health care is an enormous and lucrative industry with myriad interwoven conflicts of interest among and between stakeholders, including even the medical profession, as was documented in my recent book *The Corrosion of Medicine: Can The Profession Reclaim Its Moral Legacy?*[45] As we saw in the last chapter, the Heritage Foundation is but one of many well funded neo-conservative think tanks committed to advancing private markets through lobbying and reports that serve their interests. Its $30 million media campaign to discredit Original Medicare as an "inferior program" and "promote market solutions to the Medicare problem" illustrates its efforts to preserve the private marketplace.[46]

Enactment and implementation of NHI will require the reconstruction of responsible government independent of corporate and political influence. NHI should give us a structure for greater public accountability while the transition toward a not-for-profit health care industry should help to reduce waste and the many entrenched conflicts of interest that exist today. Our goal should be to restore public service to its rightful place and attract again the best and the brightest to government.

7. Malpractice Liability Reform

Can NHI remedy the medical malpractice problem? First, it's important to understand what the problem is, and is not. As we have already seen in Chapter 6, the costs of malpractice litigation and estimated indirect costs of defensive medicine amount to about 4 percent of our annual health care spending.[47] We often hear that skyrocketing insurance premiums are driving many good physicians out of practice and limiting patients' access to care.

A 2007 analysis of the problem by Public Citizen puts the issue in perspective. Its analysis of data in the National Practitioner Data Bank (NPDB) from 1991 to 2005 revealed that the number and total value of malpractice payments to patients have been declining since 2001; that payments are not made for frivolous claims (64 percent of payments in 2005 involved death, major or significant injuries, with less than one-third of 1 percent for "insignificant injury"); that the real problem is patient safety and preventable medical errors (eg., surgery on the wrong limb); that 82 percent of physicians have never had a medical malpractice payment since the NPDB was established in 1990; that 5.9 percent of physicians have accounted for more than one-half of medical malpractice payments since 1991; and that only one-third of physicians who had 10 or more malpractice payments were disciplined by their state board.[48] The medical malpractice issue is hyped by business interests and conservative legislators in their efforts to characterize the problem as one of frivolous claims and avoid patients' rights legislation. But the problem is more about patient safety and lack of adequate oversight at any level.

While NHI will not resolve the medical malpractice problem, it can help to address it in several important ways: (1) the 25 percent of jury awards that are devoted to paying for medical costs incurred by malpractice will be eliminated under NHI, since the government will pay physicians and hospitals that perform the corrective care;[49] (2) a National Mandatory Adverse Event Reporting system can be established; (3) hospitals can be required to use computer physician order systems, to follow Joint Commission on the Accreditation of Healthcare Organizations (JCAHO) guidelines to prevent wrong side surgery, and to limit physicians' work weeks to reduce fatigue-induced error; (4) improved regional and national oversight will be possible through a single-payer information system better revealing physicians who are outlyers from best practice standards; (5) states can be urged to strengthen their medical board governance and disciplinary roles; and (6) reimbursement for negligent physician services can be withheld.

Winners and Losers With NHI

Most parties win with NHI —first and foremost, the *raison d'être* of any health care system—patients and their families, all 300 million Americans. With one structural change to public financing, they immediately gain affordable access to all necessary health care, free choice of physician and hospital, portability and reliability of coverage. Gone are concerns about financial disaster from medical bills, the need to navigate the endless requirements of the multi-payer system, and the need to find a new physician when a private health plan changes its contracts with providers. People of all ages have access, with full dignity as insured persons, to a private delivery system with more capacity than other countries around the world.

Like all universal programs including public schooling and Social Security, this is not a welfare program. Everyone pays into it on an equitable basis. Because risks are shared across a very large single risk pool, costs can be contained even as universal coverage is assured on a sustainable basis. This is truly a public-private partnership—public financing, private health care.

Business and labor join the winners' circle, perhaps even more than they yet realize. No longer are employers held back by the increasing burden of ESI and recurrent contract disputes over health benefits. They gain the prospect of a healthier work force while in most cases paying less than they now pay for private coverage. They no longer have the administrative burden and cost of employer-sponsored insurance. They gain a level playing field in competition with international competitors in a global economy. Some 50 years ago, Walter Reuther, then national president of the United Auto Workers, saw all of this coming:[50]

> *"When American corporations reached the point where they couldn't make their business more efficient without making it less profitable, when their dependency ratios soared to unimaginable heights, when they got tens of billions behind in their health-care obligations, when the cost of carrying thousands of retirees forced them to stare bankruptcy in the face, they would come around to the idea that the markets work best when the burdens of benefits are broadly shared."*

Most physicians and other health professionals will fare much better with NHI than with today's complex private bureaucracy of multiple payers and health plans. Overhead expenses will drop overnight and paperwork simplified. With more time freed up for patient care, physicians will have more clinical autonomy as second guessing by private plan bureaucrats will end. Primary care reimbursement will increase while over-reimbursement for many specialized procedures will be reduced. For physicians and other providers, all patients will be "insured," payment will be more predictable, and they are free to compete for patients on the basis of their availability and quality of care. Charity care that can be so overwhelming as to sap the finances of physicians and hospitals will also disappear—every patient with NHI will be a paying patient.

The medical community will likely come to support NHI much sooner than the AMA and most other medical organizations expect. Although organized medicine fought against the enactment of Medicare in 1965, 90 percent of seniors were enrolled a year later, and physicians soon began to prosper with newly "insured" patients.[51] Most physicians will do well with NHI, with the exception of those drawing down high incomes for unnecessary and inappropriate services and those with ownership investments in such for-profit facilities as specialty hospitals and imaging centers.

Government gains a structure within which to better support and hold accountable a private delivery system. It will have new leverage to control surging health care costs, increase the return on health care spending, increase quality of care, and improve the population's health. A healthier population can contribute to economic growth. Resolution of the country's health care crisis can strengthen our society's social fabric and restore the public's faith in responsible government.

So who loses out with NHI? The biggest loser, of course, is the private health insurance industry. But it has had its chance to succeed—50 plus years through the employer-based and individual markets, helped along by tax exemptions and other government subsidies. As this book documents, the industry has failed the public interest, even on a playing field tilted in its favor by generous subsidies. Responsible health policy can only move on beyond an obsolete private financing system to a sustainable public financing system that better meets the nation's needs. While the huge compensation packages of insurance executives will disappear with NHI, many workers in the industry will find new job opportunities at any number of levels in the new system.

The drug, medical device, medical supply, and other health-related industries will lose their favored status to set their own prices for their products. They will have to compete the old-fashioned way—on the basis of efficacy, quality, and cost-effectiveness of their products. On the other hand, those that compete successfully can find a very large market for their products. Their shareholders will no longer realize outsized returns, but investments in these companies will become comparable to those of successful public utility companies.

Hospitals will have a mixed experience with NHI. Many hospitals will win, especially those that are for-profit. Two of five of these hospitals are already in the red. As long as they are serving community needs, they will fare better with global budgets negotiated each year as they transition to not-for-profit status. Ironically enough, "non-profit" hospitals, which account for about 60 percent of the more than 3,400 hospitals in the U. S., will face greater challenges. Though originally established to serve the poor, many have abandoned that mission and use generous tax breaks to build profit machines. According to the Congressional Budget Office, "non-profits" receive more than $12 billion a year in tax exemptions as well as the $32 billion in federal, state, and local subsidies received by the entire hospital industry each year. Many "non-profits" game the system by overstating their community benefits and maximizing their profits. As an example, Northwest Memorial is a "non-profit" in an affluent part of Cook County in Chicago. It spent less than 2 percent of its revenues on charity care in 2006 (compared to 14 percent by other hospitals in Cook County) while Gary Mecklenberg, its departing CEO, received a $16.4 million payout. These so-called "non-profits" can expect to be held much more accountable in global budget negotiations under NHI , as will investor-owned specialty hospitals and hospital chains such as HCA and Tenet.[52]

The Road Ahead:
Why Reform is Now Achievable
in a Changing Political Landscape

As is clear from the foregoing, it is long overdue to come to grips with the health crisis in this country as our health care non-system continues to fall apart. Incremental "reforms" have not worked, nor will they work in the future. We have to get on with fundamental reform, starting with establishing a single-payer public financing system.

Reform remains an educational and political issue. Resolution of this crisis will test our democracy to its core—will corporate dollars of market stakeholders continue to trump individual and public will?

The question of public financing of health care has come up on other occasions since 1912, when Teddy Roosevelt ran as a Progressive on a platform including NHI. How can we expect the outcome to be any different this time around? These factors give us optimism that a tipping point for NHI is not too far away.

1. The health care crisis continues to spread, from what was once largely a problem of the poor to the working poor, then the working middle class to today where even afflu-ent people who have insurance can be felled financially by medical bills.

2. It has become obvious to a sizable majority (close to two-thirds of the public in most polls) that fundamental reform is required, including a larger role for government.[53] A recent large national survey puts that proportion even higher. The on-line Health Care for America survey sponsored by the AFL-CIO and Working America between January 14 and March 3, 2008 involved 26,419 respondents, most of whom are insured, employed, and college graduates. Within this group, 95 percent believe that our health care system is bro-ken, needs fundamental change or should be completely re-built. More than four of five respondents think that the next generation will be worse off than today.[54]

3. Even without an economic downturn in recent years, wages are stagnant, costs of health care are increasingly unafford-able, even for the employed and insured; the nation's trade and budget deficits are worrisome, and our foreign debt exceeds previous times; consumer spending is declining as prices rise; and the threat of a recession looms that will fur-ther accelerate deterioration of our health care.

4. Wall Street is beginning to recognize the limited future of private health insurers. When the nation's largest health in-surer, Wellpoint, lowered its profit forecast on March 10, 2008 due to "higher medical costs and lower-than-expected enrollments", its shares fell by more than 16% in after-hours trading.[55] By the end of the first quarter of 2008, it joined the 52-Week Low Club with its share value at $43 compared to a 52-week high of $90. According to Sheryl Skolnick, health care analyst and senior vice president at CRT Capital Group, "it took Wellpoint imploding for us to figure out that current prices of health plans do not account

for growth in medical costs", and that in order to reverse their downturn insurers must "create affordable health insurance plans that consumers really want to buy instead of affordable-but-barebones plans that do not offer consumers a compelling value."[56]

5. The electorate is changing; Stanley Greenberg, co-founder of Democracy Corps observes that "we are entering a new period shaped by the failure of the conservative revolution, putting Democrats in a position to advance progressive ideas. Voters are abandoning conservative principles and are increasingly open to progressive values"[57] ; the Republican Party has rapidly lost public support, especially among political independents[58] ; about three in ten voters now call themselves independents, and they are likely to play a decisive role in the 2008 elections.[59]

6. Americans who have publicly financed health care like it just fine—in fact better than privately financed care—as we saw in Chapter 4 with Medicare and the VA.

7. We are seeing increasingly vigorous efforts at the state level to enact publicly-financed single-payer reform. One recent example is passage of such a bill in California only to be vetoed by Governor Schwarzenegger. With growing ferment in many states to address the health care crisis in the absence of national reform, we may see reform start in the states and spread from there to national policy, as took place in Canada after initial legislation in Saskatchewan.[60]

8. As organized labor finds its health care benefits continue to deteriorate with the decline of employer-sponsored insurance, it is becoming a stronger voice for single-payer reform, as shown by the recent endorsement of the Conyers bill (H.R. 676) by the AFL-CIO.[61]

9. Support for single-payer NHI is growing within and among the health professions as illustrated by activist positions being taken by the American College of Physicians (ACP, the second largest organization of physicians in the country with 125,000 members), Physicians for a National Health Program (PNHP), the American Public Health Association (APHA) and the California and American Nursing

Associations (CNA and ANA). A recent national survey of American physicians involving more than 2,200 respondents found that 59 percent now support single-payer NHI; of 13 specialties surveyed, all favored NHI by more than 50 percent except surgical specialists, anesthesiologists and radiologists (all three at the high reimbursement end of the spectrum).[62]

10. Publicly financed health insurance is not a new, untested idea. Almost all industrialized Western countries have one or another form of social insurance, often combined with a private delivery system. The U.S. compares poorly against many other health care systems in terms of efficiency, access, quality and equity. Although market advocates in this country like to portray NHI as a fringe idea, the opposite is the case—we are the "odd man out" around the world.

11. Although opposition to NHI will be stronger than ever as market advocates fight a rear-guard action to defend the private multi-payer system, there are more and more chinks in their armor, as noted in the last chapter. We have seen in the Preface and in later chapters how insiders within the insurance industry are more worried than ever about the industry's future. We can expect an onslaught of distortion and disinformation by opponents of NHI. But Harry and Louise won't be as effective as they were in 1994, as suggested by Figure 8.1.

At this writing (April, 2008) the outcome of the 2008 elections is not yet known. But our health care crisis, already severe, can only get worse without fundamental reform. Whichever political party controls the White House and Congress in January 2009, it cannot expect to stay in power for long without addressing this issue head-on.

NHI will not give us a perfect system. There is no such thing. But it will be a good start, and a great improvement over what we have now. The stakes are high, and getting higher each year. Table 8.5 shows how primary care and our health care system will probably look by 2020 with or without NHI.[63]

The outcome of this current debate over the future of U.S. health care will determine in large part how we view ourselves as a society—

Figure 8.1
Harry and Louise, circa 2007

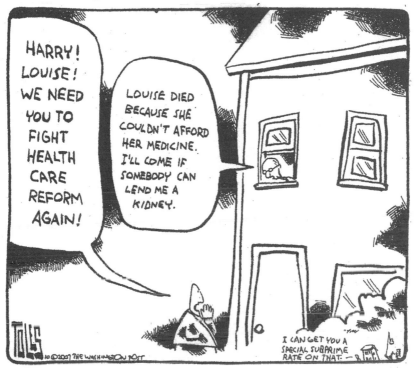

are we a united society with a sense of fair play and concern for others
matching our ideals, or a bastion of social Darwinism continuing to
pride ourselves for American exceptionalism? Based on our own experience with health care in this country and that of other industrialized
countries around the world, we already know what works, and doesn't
work, for sustainable and well-performing health care systems. The
question, as always, is what we will do about it? Ralph Nader, as the
founder of Public Citizen and one of the 100 most influential Americans in our history (and one of only 4 still living) as determined by 10
award-winning historians and authors for *The Atlantic*, reminds us of
this ancient Chinese proverb, which is as timely as timeless:

"To know and not to do is not to know."[64]

TABLE 8.5

Alternative Scenarios for 2020

Primary Care	Without NHI	With NHI
	Less in demand	More in demand
	Marginal system role	Strengthened system role
	Less continuity of care	More continuity of care
	Less well distributed	Broadly distributed
	Lower career satisfaction	Higher career satisfaction
	Marginal reimbursement	Stabilized reimbursement
	High practice overhead	Lower practice overhead
	No population-based research	Population-based research growing
	Weak primary care workforce	Larger stabilized workforce
Health Care System	Severe access problems in lower tiers	Universal access, less tiering
	Soaring cost inflation	Reasonable cost containment
	Degraded system performance	Improved system performance
	More health disparities	Improved health outcomes
	Increased public dissatisfaction	Increased patient satisfaction
	Increased bureaucracy and fragmentation	Simplified administration and less fragmented

NHI-national health insurance

Source: Adapted with permission from: Geyman JP. Drawing on the legacy of general practice to build the future of family medicine. Fam Med 36(9):631-8, 2004.

1. Archer D. Profit For Some Or Care For all. TomPaine.com February 27, 2007. Available at: http://www.tompaine.com/articles/2007/02/27/profit_for_some_or_care_for_all.php.
2. Lakoff G., Haas E., Smith G.W., & Parkinson S. *The Logic of the Health Care Debate.* Berkeley, CA: A Rockridge Institute Report. October 15, 2007. (available at www.rockridgeinstitute.org/).
3. Davis K., Schoen C., Doty M., & Tenney K. Medicare versus private insurance: Rhetoric and reality. *Health Affairs Web Exclusive* W321, October 9, 2002.
4. Geyman J. P. *The Corrosion of Medicine: Can the Profession Reclaim its*

Moral Legacy? Monroe, ME: Common Courage Press, 2008, p.

5. Himmelstein D. U. The National Health Program Slide-Show Guide. Center for National Health Program Studies. Cambridge, Mass: 2000.
6. Blue Cross and Blue Shield. Technology Evaluation Committee Reports, No. 1-28, Chicago: 1999.
7. Wolfe S. M. Selling "new" drugs using smoke and mirror (images). *Health Letter*, March 2003, pp 2-5.
8. Brownlee S. Newtered. Gingrich's Congress emasculated the one agency capable of controlling health care costs and improving quality. Time to reverse the procedure. *The Washington Monthly* 39(10):27-33, October 2007.
9. Tunis S. R. Why Medicare has not established criteria for coverage decisions. *N Engl J Med* 350(21):2196-98, 2004.
10. Diamond F. Making the case for a "Health Care Fed." *Managed Care*, January 2002:26-33.
11. Wennberg J.B., Fisher E.S. & Skinner J.S. Geography and the debate over Medicare reform. *Health Affairs Web Exclusive* W-103, February 13, 2002.
12. Goodson J.D. Unintended consequences of resource-based relative value scale reimbursement. *JAMA* 298 (19): 2308-10, 2007.
13. Bodenheimer T., Berenson R. A. & Rudolf P. The primary care specialty income gap: Why it matters. *Ann Intern Med* 146:301-6, 2007.
14. Starfield B. Is primary care essential? *Lancet* 344:1129-33, 1994.
15. The United States relies on family physicians, unlike any other specialty (Policy Center One-Pager #5). Washington, D.C.: American Academy of Family Physicians Robert Graham Center: Policy Studies in Family Practice and Primary Care, April 14, 2000.
16. Rosenblatt R.A. Specialists or generalists. On whom shall we base the American health care system? *JAMA* 267:1665-66, 1992.
17 Greenfield S., Nelson E.C., & Zubkoff M., et al. Variations in resource utilization among medical specialties and systems of care: Results from the Medical Outcomes Study. *JAMA* 267:1524-30, 1992.
18. Campbell T. L., Franks P., Fiscella K., et al. Do physicians who diagnose more mental health disorders generate lower health care costs? *J Fam Pract* 49:305-310, 2000.
19. Parchman M. & Culter S. Primary care physicians and avoidable hospitalization. *J Fam Pract* 39:123-6,1994.
20. Shi L., Starfield B., Kennedy B., & Kawachi I. Income inequality, primary care, and high indicators. *J Fam Pract* 45(4):275-84,1999.
21. Beal A.C., Doty M.M., Hernandez S.E., Shea K.K., & Davis K. Closing the divide: how medical homes promote equality in health care: results from The Commonwealth Fund 2006 Health Care Quality Survey. http://www.commonwealthfund.org/publications/publications—show. htm?doc_id=5068. Accessed June 27, 2007.
22. Bodenheimer T. Primary care—will it survive? *N Engl J Med* 355(9):861-4, 2006.
23. Woo B. Becoming a physician. Primary care—the best job in medicine? *N*

Engl J Med 355(9):864-6, 2006.

24. Rosenblatt R.A., Hart L.G., Baldwin L., Chan L. & Schneeweiss R. The generalist role of specialty physicians: is there a hidden system of primary care? *JAMA* 1998;279:1364-70 1998.

25. ACP. The impending collapse of primary care medicine and its implications for the state of the nation's health care. Washington, D.C.: American College of Physicians, January 30, 2006. (Accessed August 10, 2006, at http://www.acponline.org/hpp/statehc06_1pdf.)

26. American College of Physicians. Position Paper. Achieving a High-Performance Health Care system with Universal Access: What the United States Can Learn from Other Countries. *Ann Intern Med*, January 1, 2008.

27. AMA. Impact of increasing specialization and declining generalism in the medical profession. Reports of the American Medical Association, Council on Medical Education. www.ama-assn.org/ama1/pub/upload/mm8/a-06cme.pdf. Accessed July 24, 2007.

28. Morrison G. Mortgaging our future—the cost of medical education. *N Engl J Med* 352(2):117-9, 2005.

29. World Health Report 2000. Available at http://www.who.int/whr/000en/report.htm.

30. Schoen C., Davis K., How S..K.H. & Schoenbaum S.C. U. S. health system performance: A national scorecard. *Health Affairs Web Exclusive* W-457-W-475, 2006.

31 Banks J., Marmot M., Oldfield Z., & Smith J.P. Disease and disadvantage in the United States and in England. *JAMA* 295:2037-45, 2006.

32. Ibid #11.

33. Ibid #25.

34. Fisher E.S. & Welch H.G. Avoiding the unintended consequences of growth in medical care: How might more be worse? *JAMA* 281:446-53, 1999.

35. Davidoff F. Medicine and commerce: 1; is managed care a "monstrous hybrid"? *Ann Intern Med* 128:496-9, 1998.

36. Relman A.S. Personal communication. August 20, 2007.

37. Ibid #4, p 37.

38. Woolhandler S., Himmelstein D. U., Angell M., Young Q.D. and the Physicians Working Group for Single-Payer National Health Insurance. Proposal of the Physicians' Working Group for Single-Payer National Health Insurance. *JAMA* 290:798, 2003.

39. Lipsky M. & Stewart D. Redeeming public remedy. *The American Prospect* 18(5):A, May 2007.

40. Hartmann T. *Unequal protection: The rise of corporate dominance and the theft of human rights*. Emmaus, PA: Rodale Press, 2002, pp. 177-8.

41. Norquist G, as quoted on NPR's *Morning Edition* in May 2001.

42. Zhang, J. How government adds to ranks of uninsured. *Wall Street Journal* March 25, 2008: D1

43. Hacker J.S. *The Divided Welfare Stare: The Battle Over Public and Private Social Benefits in the United States*. Cambridge, Mass: Cambridge University

Press, 2002, p 329.

44. Reinhardt U.E. The mix of public and private payers in the U.S. health system. In: *The Public—Private Mix for Health*. Maynard A. (ed). Oxford: Seattle: Radcliffe Publishing, The Nuffield Trust, 2005: pp 110-11.

45. Ibid #4.

46. The Heritage Foundation Media Campaign. Washington, D.C.: Medicare Rights Center. http://www.medicarerights.org/maincontentheritage.html. Accessed December 1, 2003.

47. Relman A. S. *Second Opinion: Rescuing America's Health Care*. Public Affairs, New York: 2007, pp 91-2.

48. Public Citizen's analysis of malpractice payments as reported in the National Practitioner Data Bank Public Use. File for the years 1990 to 2005. Washington, D.C., January 2007.

49. Weiler P.C. Fixing the tail: the place of malpractice in health care reform. *Rutgers Law Rev*, 47:1157-92, 1995.

50. Reuther W., as cited by Gladwell M. The risk pool: What's behind Ireland's economic miracle-and GM's financial crisis? *The New Yorker*, August 28, 2006, p 35.

51. Public Citizen. Health care reform in the United States: Arguments for a single-payer system, Public Citizen's submission to the Citizen's Health Care Working Group, July 2006.

52. Carreyrou, J, Martinez, B, Nonprofit hospitals, once for the poor, strike it rich. *Wall Street Journal* , April 4, 2008: A1

53. The Health Report to the American People. Report of the Citizen's Health Care Working Group, Appendix B, July 2006, available at http://www. citizenshealthcare.gov/recommendations/appendix_b.df.

54. AFL-CIO. 2008 Health Care for America Survey. Tabulation and analysis by Peter D. Hart Research Associates. Accessed at http://www.aflcio.org/issues/healthcare/upload/healthcaresurvey.report.pdf on March 26, 2008

55. Freudenheim, M, Wellpoint cuts its outlook, sending shivers through shares of health insurers. *New York Times* , March 11, 2008: C3

56. Kaiser Daily Health Policy Report. Analysis look at first-quarter financial results of insurers for signs of industry's health. April 3, 2008.

57. Greenberg S. Democrats arc back—But---*The American Prospect* 18(7):21, July-August 2007.

58. The Pew Research Center. Trends in Political Values and Core Attitudes 1987-2007: March 22, 2007.

59. Balz D. & Cohen J. Independents' Day. A political force with many philosophies could be key in 2008 election. *The Washington Post National Weekly Edition* 24(39):11, July 16-22, 2007.

60. Armstrong P. & Armstrong H. *Universal Health Care. What the United States Can Learn from the Canadian Experience*. New York: The New Press, 1998:6-32.

61. AFL-CIO Executive Council statement. Health Care. Las Vegas, NV: March 6,

214

2007.

62. Carroll, A E, Ackermann, R T, Support for national health insurance among U. S. physicians: Five years later. *Ann Intern Med* 148: 566-7, 2008

63. Ibid #4 p 206

64. Chinese proverb, as cited by Nader R. *The Seventeen Traditions.* New York: Harper Collins, 2007, p 148.

Appendix 1

Glossary

Adverse Selection: This occurs when lower-risk individuals are split off by insurers from a larger risk pool in order to minimize their financial risk and increase these profits. The smaller risk pool of higher-risk individuals that results requires higher costs of treatment. Adverse selection is the Achilles' heel of capitation, since for-profit HMOs and some physicians are often tempted to selectively care for healthier patients.

Agency for Healthcare Research and Quality (AHRQ): This federal agency was established by Congress in 1989 as the Agency for Healthcare Policy and Research (AHCPR). Since then, its name has been changed, but its continuing activities include development of clinical practice guidelines, promotion of evidence-based medicine, reduction of medical errors, and expansion of research on the cost, utilization, and outcomes of health care.

America's Health Insurance Plans (AHIP): This is a national trade group representing about 1,300 member private insurance companies which provide coverage to about 200 million Americans. It was formed in 2003 by the merger of the American Association of Health Plans (AAHP) and the Health Insurance Association of America (HIAA).

Association Health Plans (AHPs): These are plans established by private insurers in order to better market their policies across state lines. AHPs are exempt from state rate-setting regulations in many states. Insurers claim that AHPs can make insurance more affordable for smaller employers while critics argue that AHPs allow insurers more latitude to "cherry pick" the market without assurances of adequate coverage.

Capitation: A method of payment for patient care services used by managed care organizations, such as health maintenance organizations

(HMOs), to reimburse providers under contractual agreements. Payment rates are set in advance, and are paid monthly or annually regardless of what services are actually provided to covered patients.

Carrier: Private insurers which contract with Medicare to administer supplementary health insurance under Part B of Medicare. In the earlier years, Blue Shield held most of these contracts for physician services. Today's decentralized market has many commercial insurers involved as carriers.

Center for Medicare and Medicaid Services (CMS): The federal agency which administers the Medicare program and works with the States to administer Medicaid, the State Children's Health Insurance Program (SCHIP), and health insurance portability standards. CMS accounts for 20% of the federal government's budget. In FY 2005, this amounted to about $519 billion, with nearly two-thirds of that spent on Medicare.

Disease Management: This is a new buzzword being hailed by many policy makers and legislators for its potential to rein in healthcare costs and improve the quality of care for chronic diseases such as diabetes. While effective primary care team-based disease management programs have been pioneered by not-for-profit organizations such as Group Health Cooperative and Kaiser Permanente for some years, a for-profit commercial DM industry has emerged, started by the drug industry during the 1990s, which attempts to provide patient education and improved patient self-management, mostly through nurses in distant call centers without integration with primary care.

COBRA (The Consolidated Omnibus Budget Reconciliation Act of 1985): This is the mechanism by which people who lose or change jobs which provide employer-based health insurance may regain insurance through the individual market if they can afford the premiums. Under COBRA, insurers and health plans are required to continue their previous coverage for at least 18 months.

Co-Insurance: This refers to the percentage of health care costs which are not covered by insurance and which the individual must pay. Many health insurance plans cover 80% of the costs of hospital and physician care, leaving 20% to be "self-insured" by patients receiving these services.

Community Health Centers (CHCs): These are safety net facilities and primary care practices which are intended to serve their communities regardless of ability to pay. Through federal funding and smaller public and private grants, CHCs seek to improve the health status of all members of the community, many of whom are uninsured. There are more than 1,000 CHCs located in underserved communities across the country.

Community Rating: A method for setting premiums for health insurance which is based on the average cost of health care for the covered population in a geographic area. This method shares risk across all covered individuals, whether sick or well, so that the healthy help to subsidize the care of the sick who otherwise may not be able to afford coverage on their own. As a then not-for-profit insurer, Blue Cross pioneered this method in the 1930s, but it was abandoned by most commercial insurers after the 1960s, as experience rating spread throughout the industry.

Consumer-Directed Health Care (CDHC): A strategy to contain health care costs by shifting more responsibility to consumers in choosing and paying for their own health care. Currently popular with conservatives and many moderates in government, the consumer-choice theory of cost containment assumes that there is a free market in health care, that consumers can be well informed about their choices, and that they will be more prudent in their health care decisions by taking more responsibility to pay for their costs.

Cost Effectiveness: When applied to health care, this concept attempts to estimate the value for expenditures on procedures or services that is returned to patients. Value may include longer life, better quality of life, or both. This is a complex but important area of study if affordable care of good quality is to be made available to broad populations. Cost-effectiveness analysis (CEA) is the technique used to measure costs and efficacy of alternative treatments in order to estimate their economic value, which then are typically measured in quality-adjusted life years (QALYs).

Co-Payment: Flat fee charged directly to patients whenever they seek health care services or drug prescriptions regardless of their insurance coverage. As today's trend toward consumer-directed health care gains momentum, co-payments are increasing across the health care marketplace to the point of becoming a financial barrier to care for many lower-income people.

Cost-Sharing: This term refers to requirements that patients pay directly out-of-pocket for some portion of their health care costs. The level of cost-sharing varies from one health plan to another. Although intended by insurers and many policy makers to help control the costs of health care, cost-sharing has a serious downside of discouraging many people from gaining access to necessary health care.

Death Spiral: This term is used to describe the progressive effects of adverse selection in shrinking a risk pool into a smaller population of high-risk individuals requiring expensive care. For example, as a result of "cream-skimming" by for-profit private health plans, public programs such as Medicare are placed at risk because of reduced cross subsidies from the healthy to the sick.

Deductible: Out-of-pocket costs which patients must pay before their insurance coverage kicks in for subsequent costs. This amount is required to be met each year. As policy-makers and health plans pursue the model of consumer-directed health care, deductibles and co-payment requirements of cost-sharing are increasing each year.

Defined Benefits: This term is applied when an insurance program offers a pre-determined set of benefits to all enrollees. The Medicare program is such an example, with covered benefits authorized by law.

Defined Contributions: This is the polar opposite of defined benefits. In this instance, a fixed set of benefits is not provided by the insurer, whether public or private. Instead, a defined contribution is made toward the costs of coverage (egs., by an employer or perhaps by Medicare if further privatization "reforms" are enacted) (see also Premium Support).

Distributive Justice: When used in health care, this term connotes a principle of fairness whereby health care is considered a right that should be shared within a society on the basis of need. The counter-vailing view held by proponents of an open market is that health care is a privilege that should be allocated by ability to pay. With an emphasis on markets, the U.S. is atypical from almost all other industrialized countries around the world where distributive justice is the dominant ethic underlying various systems of social health insurance.

Doughnut Hole Coverage: This is the gap between partial coverage (75%) and catastrophic coverage (95%) of the costs of prescription drugs provided to Medicare beneficiaries through the Part D Prescription Drug Benefit. The Medicare legislation of 2003 (MMA) initially set the "doughnut hole between $2,250 and $5,100 annual drug costs (a $2,850 gap) within which Medicare beneficiaries are responsible to pay these costs out-of-pocket.

Employer-Based Insurance: A voluntary system established during the wartime economy of the 1940s whereby many employers have provided health insurance overage to their employees. Today, that system is unraveling steadily, now covering only abut two-thirds of the non-elderly workforce and with many employers shifting to a defined contribution approach toward their employees' insurance costs.

Employer-Mandate: A policy considered in some states whereby all employers would be required to provide health insurance for their employees. Such a policy is usually opposed by small business, fearing costs that could put them out of business.

ERISA (Employee Retirement Income Security Act of 1974): Enacted in 1974 before the advent of managed care, ERISA was originally intended to protect pension plans, but soon became a loophole in states' attempts to regulate abuses by private health insurers. Under ERISA, all self-funded employer health plans are exempt from state regulations, as are many managed care organizations. ERISA does not apply to Medicare, Medicaid, and insurance provided by government employers.

Experience Rating: This is the current norm in U.S. health insurance markets, as opposed to the community rating tradition originally established by Blue Cross in the 1930s. Under experience rating, insurers avoid high-risk individuals and groups and increase premiums based upon illnesses experienced by enrollees. Experience rating weakens the ability of health insurance to share risk across a large risk pool of healthy and sick individuals.

Favorable Risk Selection: This is the process by which insurers screen potential enrollees according to health status, avoiding higher-risk sick individuals and groups in favor of healthier enrollees requiring less costly care (i.e., the opposite of adverse selection).

Fee-for-Service (FFS): A common method of reimbursement for health services provided, such as by visit, procedure, laboratory test or imaging study. Fees are often based on a fixed fee schedule or on more complex relative value scales.

Fiscal Intermediary: Private insurers which contract with Medicare to administer hospitalization insurance under Part A of Medicare. Blue Cross has held most of these contracts over the years. In this capacity, insurers are empowered to make coverage and reimbursement decisions and to provide related administrative services.

Formulary: Lists of drugs updated at regular intervals, which can be prescribed by physicians for enrollees in specific programs. Formularies have been developed by health plans in recent years as a means of containing escalating drug spending. Formulary development is a contentious area, with the pharmaceutical industry arguing for wider coverage lists while health plans strive to balance cost, efficacy and safety issues against patients' access to medically necessary medications.

Geographic Variation: This term is used to describe wide variations from one part of the country to another in practice patterns and services provided to Medicare beneficiaries. Regional and small area variations date back to the origins of the program, including marked differences in utilization of services as well as coverage and reimbursement policies.

Generic Drugs: Drugs which are essentially the same as their brand-name counterparts, but whose patents have expired. They are generally considerably less expensive than their brand-name equivalents.

Group Market: The private health insurance market is split into two distinct parts—group and individual markets. Group markets involve employer-based insurance, further divided into large groups and small groups. Since each state has its own regulations for the insurance industry, the overall insurance market is divided into 150 different state-level markets.

Guaranteed Issue: Typically opposed by the private insurance industry because of the potential for adverse selection, some states require insurers to provide coverage to all comers, an open-enrollment policy.

Health Care Financing Administration (HCFA): As part of the Department of Health and Human Services (DHHS), HCFA was created in 1977. It administered Medicare and Medicaid for many years until reconstituted in 2001 as the Center for Medicare and Medicaid Services (CMS).

Health Maintenance Organization (HMO): HMOs are organizations which provide a broad range of services, coordinated by primary care physicians on a prepaid basis for enrollees. First authorized by federal legislation in 1973, HMOs have developed since the 1980s to now cover about 80 million Americans. About two-thirds of HMOs are for-profit, such as Humana, while the rest are not-for-profit, such as Kaiser Permanente and Group Health of Puget Sound. HMOs vary organizationally from staff models, where physicians are salaried and work only with that HMO (egs., Kaiser and Group Health) to looser structures, such as independent practice associations (IPAs), where physicians in independent practices contract with an HMO to provide care for enrollees and are reimbursed on a capitation basis. Though it has become an imprecise term over the years, "managed care" encompasses these variations within an overall pattern of prepaid medical care.

Health Savings Account (HSA): As part of the current trend toward consumer-directed health care, health savings accounts shift more financial responsibility to consumers for the costs of their health care decisions. HSAs were authorized under the Medicare Prescription Drug, Improvement, and Modernization Act of 2003 (MMA). Employer and employee contributions are tax-free when accompanied by high deductible insurance policies. While providing new investment opportunities for healthy individuals, HSAs provide little financial protection against the costs of serious illness.

High-Deductible Health Insurance Plans (HDHI): As part of the present trend toward "consumer-directed" health care, many private insurers are offering policies with high cost-sharing requirements, including annual deductibles up to $10,000. These policies are typically associated with health savings accounts (HSAs) and provide little coverage or security for people experiencing significant medical expenses.

High-Risk Pool: With the intent to help people who have been denied coverage in the individual market to gain coverage by pooling risk with others facing the same problem, about 30 states have established high-risk pools supported by both federal and state funding. To date, however, these high-risk pools have had little success in reducing the numbers of uninsured, and their limited coverage comes with high premiums.

Individual Market: Compared to employer-sponsored health insurance covering groups of employees, the individual market is relatively small, covering only 17 million non-elderly Americans. Many applicants are denied coverage in the individual market. For those who qualify, premiums are higher and coverage less secure.

Limited-Benefit Plan: These are policies being marketed by private insurers to employers and healthier people with restricted benefits and annual caps as low as $1,000 to $2,500.

Managed Care: Although this term has often become ambiguous and unclear in common usage, it expresses a new relationship between purchasers, insurers and providers of care. To a variable extent, organizations that pay for patient care have also taken on the role of making decisions about patient care management. In practice, however, "managed care" is often more managed reimbursement than care. Three common types of managed care organizations are preferred provider organizations (PPOs), group and staff model HMOs, and independent practice association (IPA) HMOs.

Medicaid: A federal-state health insurance program, also enacted in 1965 with Medicare, which covers low-income people who meet variable and changing state eligibility requirements. Most elderly, disabled, and blind individuals who receive assistance through the federal Supplemental Security Income (SSI) program are covered under Medicaid, which is also the main payer of nursing home costs. Federal matching funds to the state range from about 50 to almost 80 percent. Current budget deficits in federal and state budgets threaten this vital safety net program, which provides last-resort coverage for about one in six Americans, including one-fifth of all children in the U.S.

Medical Loss Ratio (MLR): The medical loss ratio is that part of the premium dollar spent on direct medical care. Private insurers typically try to keep their MLR at or below 80%, retaining 20% or more of premium revenue for administrative overhead and profits.

Medical Underwriting: This is the process used by health insurers to calculate higher premiums to be charged to individual or group applicants at higher risk for illness. Medical underwriting was considered unethical in the early years of private insurance in this country, but has become the industry norm, and is usually based on annual review of claims experience.

Medigap: Private supplementary insurance which covers medical expenses not covered by Medicare, which may include co-payments, deductibles and other related costs. The rising costs of Medigap policies have led to serious underinsurance for many elderly people, with increasing out-of-pocket expenses and difficulties in affording necessary medical care. The annual costs of Medigap policies now run as high as $11,000 per year, and only one in four elderly Americans carry such coverage.

Medical Necessity: An elusive but important term which is applied to treatments and healthcare services which can be judged on the basis of clinical evidence to be effective and indicated as essential medical care. It is an ongoing challenge for health professionals, insurers, payers and policymakers to define medical necessity as part of coverage policy, made more difficult as costs are considered and as new treatments are brought into use.

Medicare: A federal insurance program for the elderly and disabled enacted in 1965 which now covers 42 million Americans with benefits including hospital care, physician and other provider services, and limited coverage of the costs of prescription drugs. Medicare beneficiaries include seniors 65 years of age and older, as well as the disabled and those with chronic kidney failure. Traditional (Original) Medicare, as the major source of coverage for one in seven Americans, pays for about one-half of beneficiaries' health care expenses, and accounts for about one-fifth of personal national health expenditures. There are four components of Medicare today:

    Part A   Hospitalization insurance
    Part B   Supplementary medical insurance
    Part C   Medicare + Choice private plans, now Medicare Advantage
    Part D   Prescription drug coverage, starting in 2006

Medicare Advantage (MA): Private health plans authorized by Medicare legislation in 2003 as the sequel to Medicare + Choice programs. Most are HMOs, though recent years have seen an increasing number of preferred provider organizations (PPOs).

Medicare + Choice (M + C): Private health plans authorized by the Balanced Budget Act of 1997 (BBA) intended by their supporters to increase choices available to Medicare beneficiaries. Most were HMOs, with other alternatives including PPOs, provider sponsored organizations (PSOs), and private fee-for-service plans (PFFS).

Medicare Prescription Drug, Improvement and Modernization Act of 2003 (MMA): Controversial legislation enacted in 2003 as the most important change in the 40-year life of Medicare. This is a very complex bill, which offers a limited prescription drug benefit while including many other elements which further privatize the program and shift more of its costs from the government to consumers. The pharmaceutical and insurance industries see far more benefits from this bill than Medicare beneficiaries themselves, and future cost projections for Medicare are already surging way beyond initial estimates.

Mental Health Parity: Insurance coverage for mental health problems extended on an equal basis with physical, biomedical disorders. The insurance industry has long been wary of such coverage, fearing high demand and adverse selection. It has opposed legislation establishing parity of mental illness, such as the Mental Health Parity Act of 1996 and all later efforts by Congress to extend such legislation.

Monopsony Purchasing: Purchasing of good and services by a single buyer, such as bulk purchasing of prescription drugs covered by the Veterans Administration using the leverage of its population to obtain discounted prices from drug manufacturers.

Moral Hazard: A concept that gained favor in the 1960s that assumes that people will overuse health care services unless they pay for them directly. Consumers can be made more prudent, the argument goes, by requiring them to pay a portion of these costs out-of-pocket. Based on this concept, together with employers' efforts to trim their exposure to their employees' health care costs, cost-sharing with consumers is increasing. There is abundant evidence, however, which discredits moral hazard as a major cause of health care inflation and recognizes the adverse effects of cost-sharing in restricting access to necessary health care for many lower-income people.

National Health Insurance (NHI): A national health insurance program that would provide universal coverage to the entire U.S. population for necessary health care. As with Medicare, NHI would be a single-payer system, government-financed with a private delivery system. Through simplified administration, such a system would provide more efficiency and cost containment than the current market-based system while offering new opportunities to improve accountability and quality assurance within the system.

Network Providers and Hospitals: This designation is used by HMOs and PPOs to indicate "preferred providers" within their network of providers and hospitals. What is often marketed by managed care organizations as preferred on the basis of quality is actually preferred on the basis of least costs. Patients are penalized by health plans by paying higher costs if they select out-of-network providers and hospitals.

Overpayment: Administratively set payments to private Medicare plans in excess of payments to traditional FFS Medicare. These are provided as incentives to bring in and retain more private plans in the Medicare program. Overpayments belie the notion that private plans save money. Overpayments vary widely around the country, now averaging 112% for Medicare Advantage and ranging up to 132% of FFS Medicare in some high-cost counties.

Part D Prescription Drug Benefit: Part D is a new component of the Medicare program established in Medicare legislation of 2003 (MMA) whereby partial coverage of prescription drug expenses are provided to Medicare beneficiaries through the private sector.

Pay-for-Performance (P4P): P4P initiatives are now in progress among some health plans and as a Medicare demonstration program to test whether reimbursement incentives can result in improved quality of patient care. The jury is still out on the effectiveness of this approach toward quality improvement.

Point of Service (POS): Hybrid health plans developed by insurers to give enrollees more choice of providers than provided in conventional HMO plans. Under a POS plan, enrollees are permitted to seek out-of-network care by paying the additional costs out-of-pocket.

Pre-Existing Condition: In the process of medical underwriting as insurers evaluate applicants for coverage, medical conditions which pre-date the application are scrutinized as they relate to future health risks. They may be used to deny coverage or to raise initial premiums; if coverage is offered, insurers typically require a six-month waiting period before enrollment.

Preferred Provider Organization (PPO): An increasingly popular kind of health plan developed in reaction to many patients' resistance to being locked-in to limited panels of providers. Providers in a PPO panel agree to accept set discounted fees in exchange for the practice-building opportunity of being listed as a "preferred provider."

Premium Support: This is a strategy being promoted by some in an effort to limit the government's financial responsibility to Medicare beneficiaries by shifting from a defined benefit program to a defined contribution approach. Under premium support, the government would pay a set amount toward the cost of a plan, whether FFS, HMO or PPO, with enrollees responsible for any price differences. First proposed in the mid-1990s, the premium support concept remains controversial, including the extent to which it could save the government money.

Pre-Paid Group Practice: The concept of pre-payment for health care on a monthly or annual basis was pioneered by Henry Kaiser's non-for-profit HMO during World War II, followed a few years later by another staff-model HMO, Group Health of Puget Sound. Future costs of comprehensive care of patients covered in this way thereby became predictable while salaried participating physicians were not motivated to provide inappropriate or unnecessary services as may happen with fee-for-service reimbursement.

Provider Sponsored Organization (PSO): Another kind of managed care organization which can contract with Medicare as a Part C participating private plan under federal legislation passed in 1997. PSOs are organizations of hospitals, physician groups, or combinations thereof, which bear some financial risk for providing covered services.

Resource-Based Relative Value Scale (RBRVS): Under this system, fees for physicians are set for each service by estimating such factors as time, mental effort and judgment, and technical skill involved in each service. RBRVS was adopted by Medicare in the early 1990s in an effort to reduce the wide disparities in reimbursement of procedure-oriented specialists and primary care physicians.

Risk Adjustment: A complex technical process intended to estimate the difference in health status and risk in populations enrolled in Medicare private plans compared to FFS Medicare. It is well documented that private plans attract healthier patients requiring less costly care than Original Medicare through favorable risk selection. Risk adjustment techniques so far have been too crude to deal effectively with this problem and have been strongly resisted by private plans.

Risk Pool: A group of people considered together in order to price their insurance coverage. The larger and more diverse the group in terms of health status, the more effective insurance can be in having healthier individuals share the higher costs of care of sicker individuals while assuring the most affordable insurance premiums for the entire group.

Quality Assurance: A broad field which has developed in recent years with the goal to improve the quality of clinical practice, reduce the rate of medical errors, and improve patient care outcomes. This is an ongoing and difficult challenge, with evidence-based clinical practice guidelines an integral part of the process.

Socialized Medicine: Socialized medicine refers to a publicly-financed government owned and operated delivery system. The National Health Service in England is such an example, with government ownership of hospitals and physicians as salaried public employees. A system of publicly-financed social insurance, such as Medicare, coupled as it is with a private delivery system, is in no way socialized medicine.

State Children's Health Insurance Program (SCHIP): A federal health insurance program enacted in 1997 as a companion program to Medicaid. SCHIP was initially intended to cover uninsured children in families with incomes at or below 200% of the federal poverty level ($41,300 for a family of four in 2007) but above the traditional income eligibility level for Medicaid. There is wide variation from state to state in these eligibility levels.

Selective Contracting: A change during the 1980s when many purchasers and insurers chose to contract selectively with physicians and hospitals, deciding which providers they would pay and which they would not pay. This was intended to hold costs down, and has significantly changed the power relationships among these parties.

Single-payer: One health care financing system covering an entire population on the basis of social insurance and replacing a multipayer system of private insurance. The Medicare program in the U.S. is one such program for the elderly and disabled. Other industrialized countries around the world have their whole populations covered under one or another form of universal health insurance. The U.S. has had such bills put forward in Congress on a number of occasions, including H.R. 676 in the House today, but so far there has not been the political will to overcome the resistance of private stakeholders in our current market-based system.

Social Insurance: Social insurance is compulsory, usually provided by a public agency, and spreads the financial risk of illness across an entire population, making its costs affordable to a large population. This is in marked contrast to private insurance, which is voluntary, provided by private insurers (usually for-profit) which selectively enroll better risks, thereby rendering coverage unaffordable or otherwise unavailable to higher-risk individuals. Medicare over the last 40 years has been a social insurance program, but it is threatened by further privatization.

Take-Up Rates: These are the rates at which employees accept health insurance coverage by their employers. Recent years have seen more restrictive eligibility policies and higher cost-sharing with employees, so that take-up rates can be quite low as coverage becomes less affordable.

Tiered Cost-Sharing: Tiered cost-sharing refers to multiple levels of cost sharing for some services, such as certain kinds of hospitals or some kinds of prescription drugs. For more expensive services or drugs, enrollees are required to pay more, either in higher co-payments and/or higher out-of-pocket costs. As an example, drug formularies for some health plans may encourage enrollees to use generic and formulary drugs by setting higher levels of cost-sharing for brand-name and non-formulary drugs.

Underinsurance: As the costs of health care continue to rise at rates several times the rates of cost-of-living and median family incomes, fewer people can afford insurance with comprehensive benefits. If they can afford coverage at all, they find themselves challenged by high levels of cost-sharing. The Commonwealth Fund has recently defined underinsurance on the basis of the proportion of total family income spent on health care (ie., more than 10% of income, more than 5% of income if below 200% of federal poverty level, or deductibles equal to or exceeding 5% of income).

Uninsurance: This term refers to the growing number, now some 47 million Americans, who have no health insurance, whether private or public. This is a large and heterogeneous group, about one in six of our population. A majority of the uninsured are employed but without affordable coverage or in part-time work without benefits. Many uninsured lose coverage with a recent job change, divorce, or death of a previously insured spouse. Many other uninsured do not qualify for public safety net programs such as Medicaid and SCHIP.

Universal Coverage: This term is used to describe countries which provide health insurance to all citizens regardless of age, income, or health status. The U.S. is atypical in not having universal coverage, as illustrated by one in six Americans being uninsured and tens of millions underinsured.

Utilization Management (UM): A cost containment strategy used by Medicare and Medicaid for many years, and more recently adopted by private health plans. Under utilization management, the clinical activities of physicians are monitored and payment for some services are denied if considered by the payer to be unnecessary. Critics of this approach contend that UM is an unwarranted intrusion into the physician-patient relationship, involves a burdensome administrative hassle for caregivers, and doesn't save much money anyway.

Voucher: A grant of money for a specific purpose, such as for meals. The idea of vouchers has been raised by supporters of premium support for Medicare, which would change the program from one of defined benefits guaranteed by the government to one of defined contributions by the government to Medicare beneficiaries. Critics see this approach as a threat to the integrity and viability of the Medicare program, by also opening the door to stepwise future reductions in the level of government contributions.

Appendix 2

Federal Poverty Guidelines, 2007
Federal Poverty Level (FPL)

Family Size in 48 Contiguous States	100 %FPL	200% FPL	300% FPL
1 person	$10,210	$20,420	$30,630
2 persons	$13,690	$27,380	$41,070
3 persons	$17,170	$34,340	$51,510
4 persons	$20,650	$41,300	$61,950

Source: DHHS, 2007

Appendix 3

H.R. 676, "The United States National Health Insurance Act," Or "Expanded & Improved Medicare For All" Introduced by Rep. John Conyers, Jr.

Brief Summary of Legislation

The United States National Health Insurance Act (USNHI) establishes a unique American universal health insurance program with single payer financing. The bill would create a publicly financed, privately delivered health care system that improves and expands the already existing Medicare program to all U.S. residents, and all residents living in U.S. territories. The goal of the legislation is to ensure that all Americans will have access, guaranteed by law, to the highest quality and most cost effective health care services regardless of their employment, income or health care status. With 47 million uninsured Americans, and another 50 million who are underinsured, the time has come to change our inefficient and costly fragmented non-system of health care.

Who is Eligible

Every person living or visiting in the United States and the U.S. Territories would receive a United States National Health Insurance Card and ID number once they enroll at the appropriate location. Social Security numbers may not be used when assigning ID cards.

Health Care Services Covered

This program will cover all medically necessary services, including primary care, inpatient care, outpatient care, emergency care, prescription drugs, durable medical equipment, hearing services, long term care, mental health services, dentistry, eye care, chiropractic, and substance abuse treatment. Patients have their choice of physicians, providers, hospitals, clinics, and practices. No co-pays or deductibles are permissible under this act.

Conversion To A Non-Profit Health Care System

Private health insurers shall be prohibited under this act from selling coverage that duplicates the benefits of the USNHI program. Exceptions to this rule include coverage for cosmetic surgery, and other medically unnecessary treatments. Those who are displaced as the result of the transition to a non-profit health care system are the first to be hired and retrained under this act. Those not rehired would receive 2 years unemployment benefits. The conversion to a not-for-profit health care system will take place over a 15 year period, through the sale of U.S. treasury bonds.

Cost Containment Provisions/ Reimbursement

The USNHI program will negotiate reimbursement rates annually with physicians, allow for global budgets (monthly lump sums for operating expenses) for hospitals, and negotiate prices for prescription drugs, medical supplies and equipment. A "Medicare For All Trust Fund" will be established to ensure a dedicated stream of funding. An annual appropriation is also authorized to ensure optimal levels of funding for the program

H.R. 676 Would Reduce Overall Health Care Costs

Families Will Pay Less

Currently, the average family of four covered under an employee health plan spends a total of $4,225 on health care annually – $2,713 on premiums and another $1,522 on medical services, drugs and supplies (Employer Health Benefits 2006 Annual Survey, Kaiser Family Foundation and Health Research and Educational Trust; U.S. Department of Labor, Bureau of Labor Statistics, Consumer Expenditure Survey.) This figure does not include the additional 1.45% Medicare payroll tax levied on employees. A study by Dean Baker of the Center for Economic Research and Policy concluded that under H.R. 676, a family of four making the median family income of $56,200 per year would pay about $2,700 for all health care costs.

Business Will Pay Less

In 2006, health insurers charged employers an average of $11,500 for a health plan for a family of four. On average, the employer paid 74% of this premium, or $8,510 per year. This figure does not include the additional 1.45% payroll tax levied on employers for Medicare. Under H.R. 676, employers would pay a 4.75% payroll tax for all health care costs. For an employee making the median family income of $56,200 per year, the employer would pay about $2,700.

The Nation Will Pay About the Same, While Covering All Americans

Savings from reduced administration, bulk purchasing, and coordination among providers will allow coverage for all Americans while reducing health care inflation in the long term. Annual savings from enacting H.R. 676 are estimated at $387 billion (Baker).

Proposed Funding For USNHI Program

- Maintain current federal and state funding for existing health care programs
- Establish employer/employee payroll tax of 4.75% (includes present 1.45% Medicare tax)
- Establish a 5% health tax on the top 5% of income earners, 10% tax on top 1% of wage earners
- 1/4 of 1% stock transaction tax
- Close corporate tax loopholes
- Repeal the Bush tax cuts for the highest income earners

For more information, contact Joel Segal (joel.segal@mail.house.gov) or Alexia Smokler (alexia.smokler@mail.house.gov) with Rep. John Conyers at 202 225-5126, or contact Olivia Boykins at 313 961-5670.

Index

About the Author

John Geyman, MD is Professor Emeritus of Family Medicine at the University of Washington School of Medicine in Seattle, where he served as Chairman of the Department of Family Medicine from 1976 to 1990. As a family physician with over 25 years in academic medicine, he has also practiced in rural communities for 13 years. He was the founding editor of *The Journal of Family Practice* (1973 to 1990) and the editor of *The Journal of the American Board of Family Practice* from 1990 to 2003. His most recent books are *Health Care in America: Can Our Ailing System Be Healed?* (Butterworth-Heinemann, 2002), *The Corporate Transformation of Health Care: Can the Public Interest Still Be Served?* (Springer Publishing Company, 2004), *Falling Through the Safety Net: Americans Without Health Insurance* (Common Courage Press, 2005), *Shredding the Social Contract: The Privatization of Medicare* (Common Courage Press, 2006), and *The Corrosion of Medicine: Can the Profession Reclaim its Moral Legacy?* (Common Courage Press, 2008), Dr. Geyman served as President of Physicians for a National Health Program from 2005 to 2007 and is a member of the Institute of Medicine.

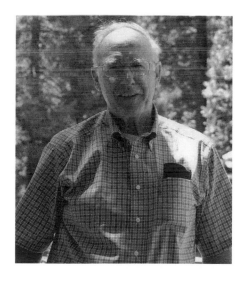